"It is a must-have for parents and grandparents alike."

—VICTORIA MCEVOY, M.D., Assistant Professor of Pediatrics at Harvard Medical School and Medical Director and Chief of Pediatrics at Massachusetts General West Medical Group

"This well-written and highly attractive book surpasses the traditional expert advice on the nutritional content and preparation of healthy foods by invoking a developmental approach to infant nutrition. In addition to learning about healthy food selection and preparation, the reader is introduced to such developmental landmarks as the infant's readiness to start solids and to begin to familiarize with spoon feeding and the tastes and textures of various foods, and the emergence of such skills as swallowing and chewing. Descriptions of subtle behavioral cues of feeding readiness, such as the infant leaning towards a spoonful of solid food, provide a clear and sound rationale for nutritional recommendations. Cogent explanations of the role of nutrients such as fat and vitamins in infant physiology inform the selection of healthy foods. The reader will not only learn how simple it is to make their baby's meals at home, but also understand the developmental and physiological rationales for healthy food choices. This is anticipatory guidance on infant nutrition at its best!"

—PAUL H. DWORKIN, M.D., Professor and Chair of Pediatrics at the University of Connecticut School of Medicine and Physician-in-Chief of the Connecticut Children's Medical Center

"As the obesity epidemic spreads across the world and parents become more concerned than ever with what to put in their children's mouths, *The Best Homemade Baby Food on the Planet* takes a lot of the guesswork and frustration out of this important parenting task. It is a must-have for parents and grandparents alike."

—VICTORIA MCEVOY, M.D., Assistant Professor of Pediatrics at Harvard Medical School and Medical Director and Chief of Pediatrics at Massachusetts General West Medical Group

"Tina Ruggiero and Karin Knight have compiled an amazingly beautiful cookbook that shows you how easy it is to make healthy and attractive food for even the pickiest of little ones. *The Best Homemade Baby Food on the Planet* guides you through the first foods to finger foods and beyond with style and ease."

—ROBIN ELISE WEISS, L.C.C.E., C.L.C., mother of eight and author of *The Complete Illustrated Pregnancy Companion* and *The Better Way to Breastfeed*

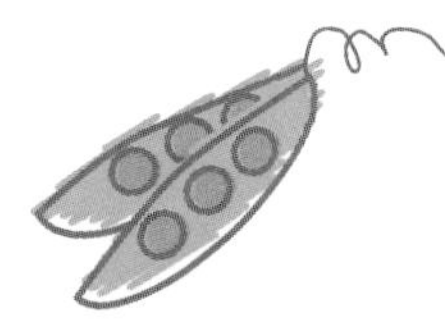

First published in the USA in 2010 by
Fair Winds Press, a member of
Quarto Publishing Group USA Inc.
100 Cummings Center
Suite 406-L
Beverly, MA 01915-6101
www.fairwindspress.com

15 14 18

ISBN-13: 978-1-59233-423-0
ISBN-10: 1-59233-423-7

Library of Congress Cataloging-in-Publication Data available

Book design: carol holtz | holtzdesign.com
Food photography: Ekaterina Smirnova
Food Styling: Travis Grandon
Prop Styling: Lauren Niles
Photographer credits: © Food Collection/agefotostock.com, 189, Jade Gedeon, 10; 40, Charles Gullung/gettyimages.com, 20, iStockphoto.com, 4; 95; 120, © Juice Images/agefotostock.com, 206, © Beverly Logan/agefotostock.com, 172, © Don Mason/agefotostock.com, 109, Move Art Management/agefotostock.com, 156, © Jose Luis Pelaez Inc/agefotostock.com, 184; 218, Andersen Ross/gettyimages.com, cover & 26; 66, sot/gettyimages.com, 93, Thinkstock, 9, Rebecca Webb, 125
Illustrations: iStockphoto.com
Photo props on pages 14, 45, 57 (spoon), 111 (fork), and 117 provided by Beaba, www.beaba.com. (Note: All Beaba products are BPA-free.)

Printed and bound in China

THE BEST HOMEMADE BABY FOOD ON THE PLANET

Know What Goes into Every Bite with
More than 200 of the Most Deliciously Nutritious
Homemade Baby Food Recipes

Karin Knight, R.N.
Tina Ruggiero, M.S., R.D., L.D.

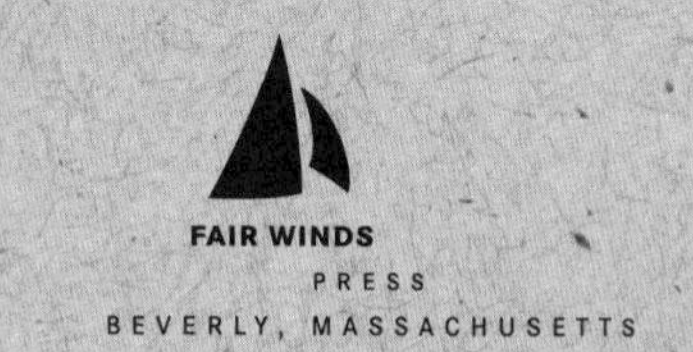
FAIR WINDS
PRESS
BEVERLY, MASSACHUSETTS

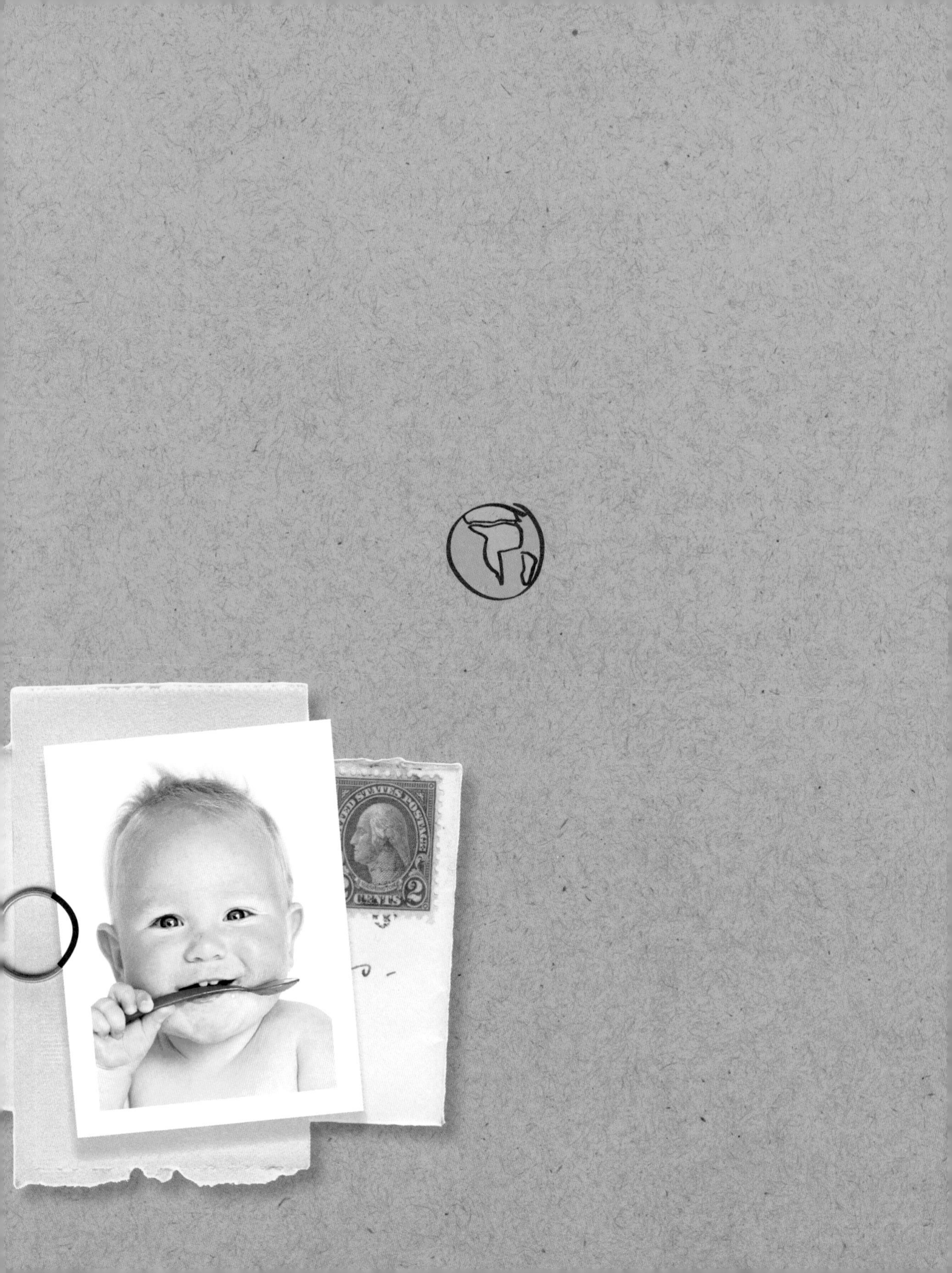

To Jody and Robert
—Karin Knight

For Mom and Dad with love
—Tina Ruggiero

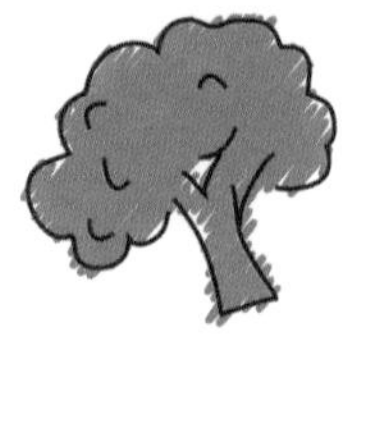

Contents

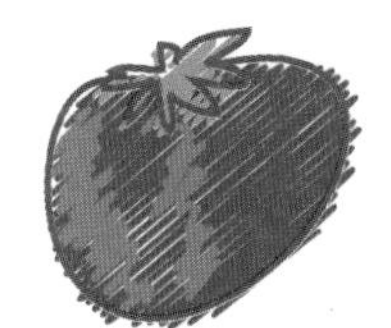

INTRODUCTION

High-Fives from the High Chair

In an era where everything is fast—from the food we eat to the pace we keep—you might think it's impossible to make your own baby food, but this book will show you how in surprisingly simple ways that save you time, effort, and money.

This book was written for every parent who wants to give their child the gift of healthy eating habits that will last a lifetime. For parents, grandparents, and other caregivers, *The Best Homemade Baby Food on the Planet* will become your trusted resource when it comes to feeding infants and toddlers. Each recipe has been professionally tested and baby approved, and most can be made in less than 10 minutes.

The recipes use common ingredients that you probably have on hand, and many can be safely refrigerated for a few days or frozen for later use. Some don't even require cooking! Best of all, the recipes in this book have significant nutrient value and will help babies and toddlers develop a well-rounded palate that's essential to establishing preferences for vegetables, fruit, and other "superfoods" important for proper growth and development.

Given the health issues beginning to plague very young children—from obesity to type 2 diabetes—it's imperative that parents introduce infants to nourishing, high-quality foods from the outset since doing so will help shape a child's food preferences and positively impact them for life. This book seeks to help you on this path by providing you with delectable, straightforward recipes that are perfectly portioned for the healthy baby and toddler. No matter which recipes you prepare, each offers taste, nutrition, simplicity, and enjoyment.

Take out your blender, feeding spoon, and baby bib and get ready for a fun-filled adventure with your little one. There are many tasty memories ahead!

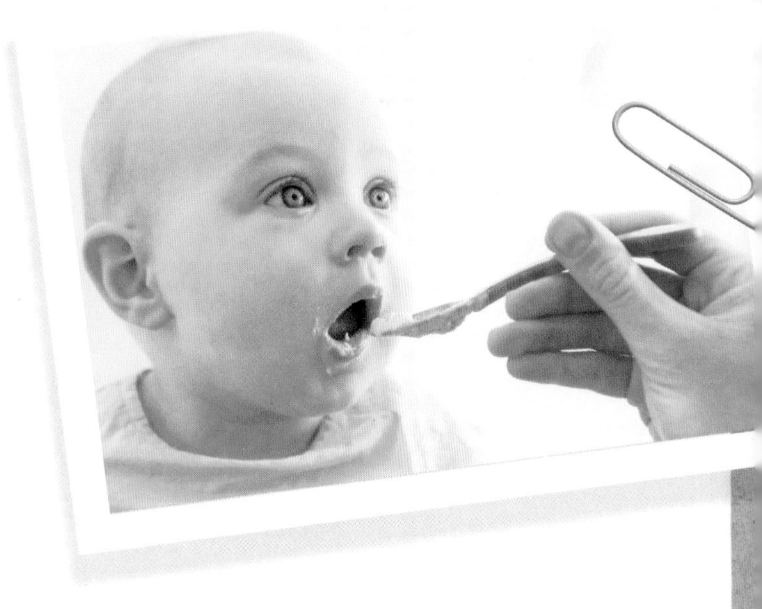

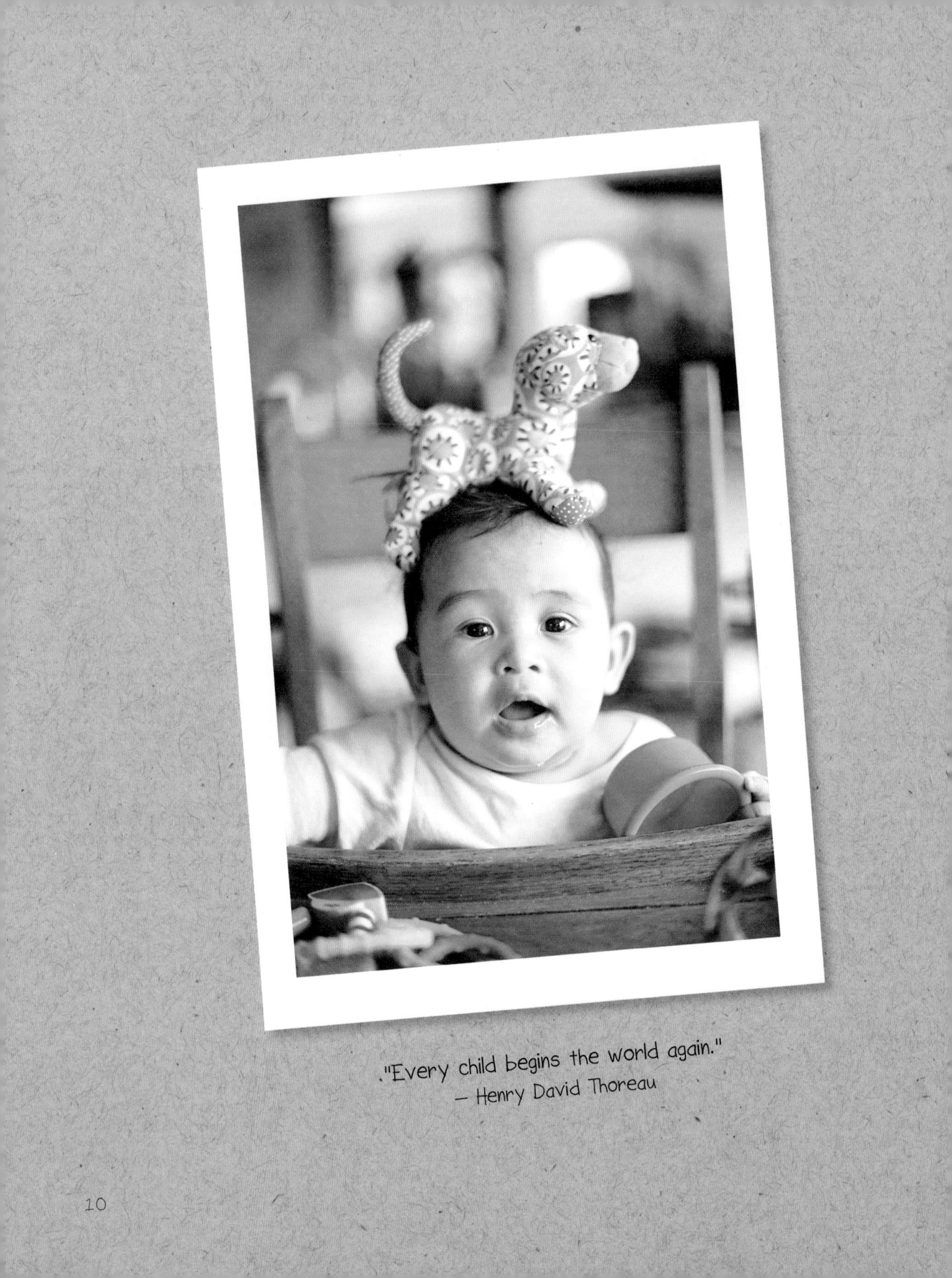

"Every child begins the world again."
— Henry David Thoreau

CHAPTER ONE

1, 2, 3, Homemade:
Your Pure and Simple Guide to Making the Best Baby Food on the Planet

While it might sound complicated, making your own baby food is really quite simple. You don't need special skills, lots of time, or expensive produce. All you need are fresh ingredients and a few simple tools. By following our suggestions on the next several pages, you'll be a pro in no time, and your baby's first meals will be an exciting and enjoyable experience for both of you!

Homemade vs. Store-Bought Baby Food: Why Homemade Is Best

There's nothing like the taste of fresh, homemade baby food. And there's no doubt it's more nutritious than the commercially prepared varieties. Why? Because the ingredients used to make ready-made baby foods are heated to very high temperatures to sterilize them and to extend their shelf life. While this makes the food safe for baby and convenient for you, the process also destroys most of the natural flavors and aromas and even worse, some of the key nutrients. See for yourself; compare the homemade purées in this book with the commercial brands you find in your local grocery store. You'll be amazed by the difference.

You'll also find that making your own baby food can be less expensive than buying prepared jars of food, and that blending and freezing batches of purées will save you precious time in the long run. Most important, by introducing your baby to pure and wholesome ingredients at this tender age, you'll be preparing him for a lifetime of healthy eating.

The goal of this book is to show you just how simple it can be to make your baby's meals at home; it's really not as time-consuming as you think! And once you've begun to make and freeze different types of meals, you'll have your own special stock to choose from, and running out of anything won't ever be a concern. Sound simple? That's because it is!

Tasty Success in 10 Minutes or Less!

Many of the baby recipes in this book can be prepared on the stovetop, in the oven, or in the microwave, and most can be made in 10 minutes or less. Some recipes don't even require cooking at all! Wherever possible, all methods of cooking are listed.

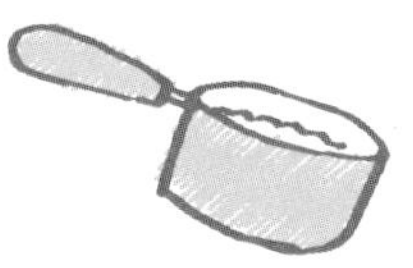

Should You Go Organic or Not?

During the past several years, interest in organic food has soared. Organic baby food, in particular, has grown in popularity as parents have become more concerned about the potential effects pesticide residues might have on their baby's health.

The most basic definition of organically grown food is that it is produced without the addition of synthetic chemicals—including fertilizers, pesticides, herbicides, and fungicides—and without the addition of hormones such as bovine growth hormone and antibiotics. It has also not been genetically engineered. To carry the official "organic" label in the United States, food must be grown according to a set of uniform standards approved by the U.S. Department of Agriculture (USDA). But does an organic seal mean that a food tastes better or is more nutritious than something that's been traditionally grown? Not necessarily, and that's why you shouldn't feel that a non-organic diet is unhealthy.

Currently, science can't tell us whether organic foods are more nutritious than non-organic ones, so if buying organic foods is cost prohibitive, you shouldn't feel guilty. Just by making your baby's meals from scratch, you're giving her a tremendous advantage in life, and your efforts should be applauded! Likewise, if organic is your way of life or if you'd like to just try incorporating some organically grown foods into your baby's diet, more power to you.

If you do plan on buying some organic ingredients to incorporate into your baby's meals, our advice is to first focus on purchasing the organic counterparts of produce that are most heavily treated with pesticides (see list below). Reason being, children are at greater risk from pesticide residues than adults because they typically eat more produce per pound of body weight than adults do.

Based on research from the USDA and the Food and Drug Administration, the Environmental Working Group has ranked produce by its pesticide content, from highest to lowest. So when grocery shopping, it's best to buy organic varieties of the following foods:

- Peaches
- Apples
- Sweet Bell Peppers
- Celery
- Nectarines
- Blueberries
- Strawberries
- Cherries
- Kale/Collard Greens
- Potatoes
- Imported Grapes
- Spinach

Your Stress-Free Start Guide: What You'll Need

You probably have most of the items you'll need to make your own baby food on hand already. Simple equipment works best. Many times, infant and toddler foods can be made with just a fork or spoon. And while the recipes in this book were tested with a simple, three-speed blender, alternatives for puréeing include baby food cookers, food mills, and baby food grinders. (Food processors don't deliver the best results, since you're working with very small amounts of ingredients.) If a purée needs thinning, use breast milk, formula, or water.

Finally, while it's important to sterilize baby bottles and nipples until your baby is 1 year old, it is not necessary to sterilize the equipment you use for food preparation. You won't need to sterilize weaning spoons or bowls either, but it's essential that you wash them well in hot, soapy water; milk used to thin purées is the ideal breeding ground for bacteria.

Here is a list of basic equipment you'll want to have on hand:

- Baby food grinder, cooker, food mill, hand-held blender, or standard blender
- Chopping knife
- Feeding cup
- Ice cube trays with covers
- Instant-read meat thermometer
- Kitchen scissors
- Measuring spoons and cups
- Microwave-safe glass bowls and lids in various sizes*
- Oven- and microwave-safe baking dishes*
- Paring knife
- Plastic or tempered glass cutting boards (dishwasher safe)
- Potato masher
- Rubber spatula
- Small covered containers for leftovers
- Small and medium size frying pans with lids
- Small and medium size saucepans with lids
- Small sieve or strainer
- Timer
- Vegetable brush (should be dishwater safe)
- Vegetable peeler
- Weaning bowl (with or without suction cups)
- Weaning spoon

* When you use the microwave, always use microwave-safe dishes and use a glass lid or plate as a cover instead of plastic or plastic wrap, which could leach chemicals into the food. Parchment paper is also safe. Never use metal or tinfoil in the microwave. Use an oven mitt or towel when removing dishes from the microwave oven to prevent burns. Microwave directions in these recipes are based on an 800-watt oven.

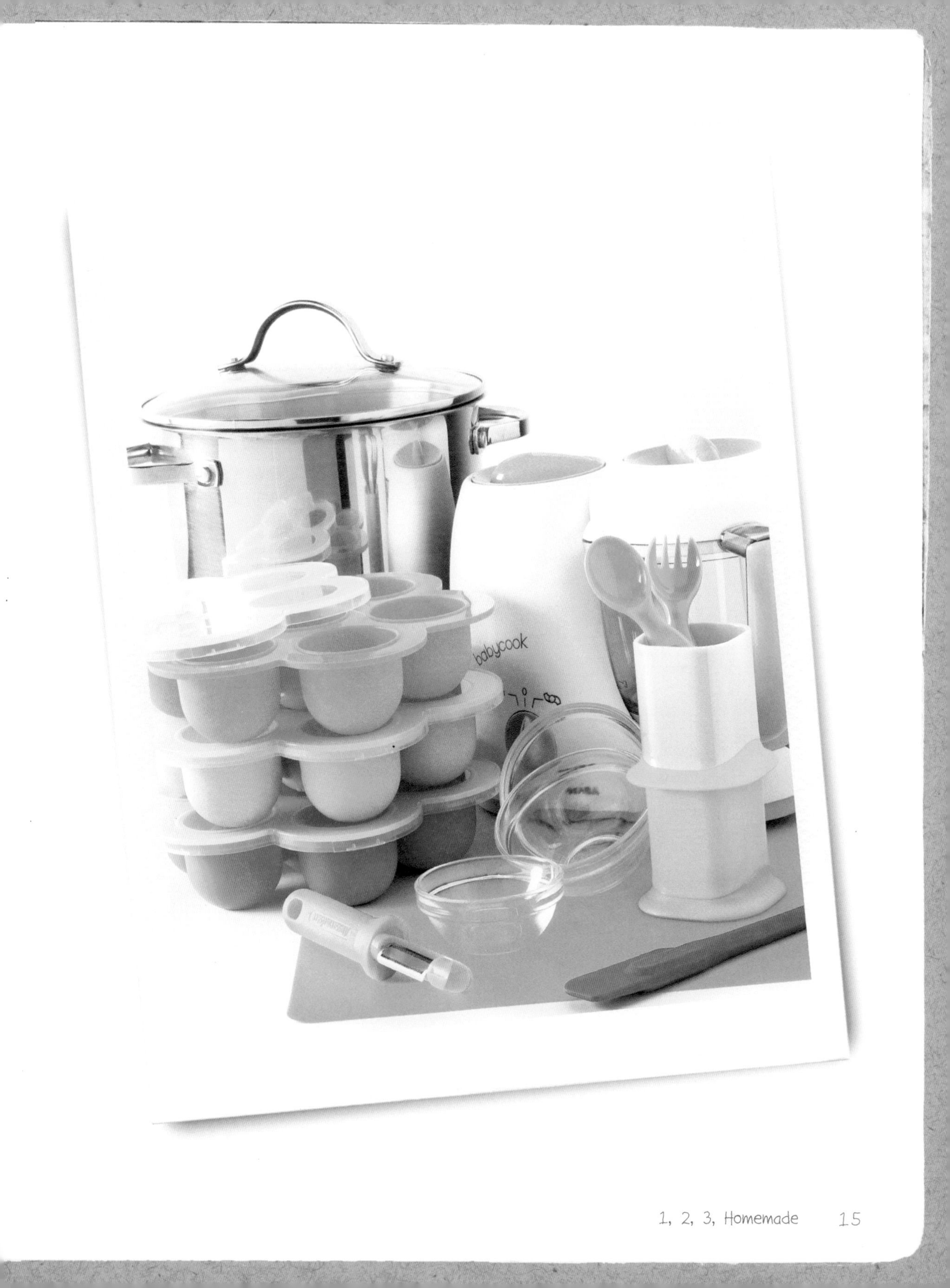
babycook

Stocking a Healthy Pantry

The key to being able to prepare healthy meals with ease and speed is to have a well-stocked pantry. Below is a comprehensive list to help you get started—you may not need all of these items from the onset, but most of them store very well, so if you have the space, stock up.

Once you have the items below on hand—along with some fresh staples like eggs, whole milk, plain yogurt, unsalted butter, and your family's favorite unprocessed cheeses—cooking any item in this book, or even preparing a healthy meal for your family, will be stress-free and enjoyable.

Here is a list of pantry staples for baby and family:

- Unsweetened applesauce
- Beans and legumes
- Canned tuna
- Canned, no sugar added fruit nectar (pear, mango, papaya, etc.)
- Assorted, unsulphured dried fruit
- Frozen vegetables (broccoli, spinach, corn, peas, carrots, vegetable blend, etc.)
- Good quality natural pasta sauce (no sugar added)
- Low-sugar whole grain cereal
- Natural chicken broth
- Oatmeal, brown rice, barley, bulgar and other whole grains
- Olive oil*
- Peanut butter, almond butter, or any other nut butter
- Pumpkin (100% pure, canned)
- Whole grain pasta

* When using oil in cooking for baby, choose regular olive oil unless extra-virgin olive oil or other oils are suggested. The taste is milder.

USING FULL-FAT DAIRY PRODUCTS

When it comes to dairy products for your baby, don't skip on the fat. Fat and cholesterol are important nutrients in your baby's diet and essential for proper growth and development. Fat is essential to absorb vitamins A, E, D, and K.

While full-fat is recommended for milk, yogurt, and other dairy products, additives are not. This means that your butter should be unsalted, and your yogurt should be plain. Be sure the yogurt is not sweetened with honey, and do not mistake vanilla yogurt for plain yogurt; they should not be used interchangeably in these recipes. Vanilla yogurt has a high sugar content and should only be used as a sweetener in moderation. Whole-milk yogurt is preferable since, again, dietary fat is critical to a baby's growth and development.

Read Before You Proceed: Ten Important Food Safety Tips

Infants are vulnerable to food-borne illnesses, so it's important you take precautionary measures when preparing homemade baby food. Just a little knowledge of food safety will go a long way to keeping your baby healthy.

1. **Wash your hands thoroughly** with hot, soapy water before preparation and in between handling raw and cooked food. Wash all surfaces, boards, and utensils with hot soapy water and rinse them well. Take apart food grinders, blenders, and baby food cookers after each use and wash thoroughly. Dry each part with a clean, dry cloth or disposable paper towels before putting appliances back together.
2. **Use fresh, high-quality food** that has been stored in clean containers at correct refrigerator temperatures (between 35°F and 38°F [1.7°C to 3.3°C]). Fresh fruits and vegetables should be used within a few days of purchase to preserve the vitamins; root vegetables can be stored for at least one week.
3. **Wash, scrub, or peel all fruits and vegetables.** Remove seeds and pits.
4. **Rinse fish, meat (except ground meats), and poultry before preparing.** Remove skin, bones, gristle, fat, and connective tissue. Use a separate cutting board for all meats.
5. **Grind tough food, seeds, and nuts.** Purée, mash, or cut food into small pieces appropriate to your baby's age and use breast milk, formula or water to thin food to the desired consistency.
6. **Microwave, steam, stir-fry, bake, broil, or roast food for optimum nutrition.** Try to avoid boiling, as this method allows nutrients to leach into the water. If you do need to boil, use as little water as possible and save the cooking water for thinning purées or in soups.
7. **Cook ground meat to a temperature of at least 165°F (74°C),** so it's no longer pink but uniformly brown throughout ("medium"). Use an instant-read meat thermometer.
8. **Do not add salt, pepper, sugar, or sweeteners to your baby's food.** Instead, season with puréed fruit or fruit juice. At one year, you can begin using herbs and spices.
9. **Discard leftover food in baby's dish after a meal.** However, leftovers from the pan or serving dish can be put in clean, covered containers and refrigerated immediately. Refrigerated leftovers should be eaten within three to four days.
10. **An infant's mouth is much more sensitive to heat than an adult's, so be cautious when serving your baby freshly heated or cooked foods**. Be sure that the food is lukewarm or room temperature and test it first by tasting a little bit yourself.

Kitchen Shortcut: Batch-Cook and Freeze!

Since preparing small amounts of purées can be time consuming, we highly recommend batch cooking as a way to save time and keep your baby's meals varied. If you're not already familiar with the concept, batch cooking involves preparing several different recipes at once, often in doubled or tripled amounts, and then freezing the extra portions. To give batch cooking a try (for your baby or your whole family) do the following:

1. **Plan what day your batch cooking will take place.** Many people choose to do this on Sundays when they have more time to spend at the stove.
2. **Select three or four recipes you'd like to make** on that day and double or triple them, noting the adjusted amounts in the recipe margin or on a sheet of paper. The majority of the recipes in this book can easily be doubled or tripled with hardly any math at all.
3. **Create a shopping list of everything you'll need.** Complete the shopping in advance.
4. **When your cooking day arrives, start with processes that will take the longest** (such as cooking brown rice or peeling vegetables) and work your way through the recipes as you see fit.
5. **Once your meals have cooled to room temperature,** refrigerate what you'll be able to use in the next two days and freeze the rest (be sure to label with contents and date). Purées can be placed in ice cube trays with covers; make sure the trays are clean and dry before using. (For more information on freezing, see the following page.)

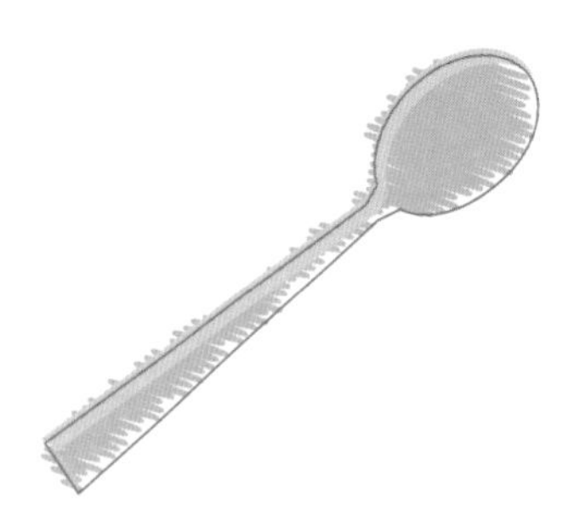

THE SAFEST WAY TO FREEZE BABY FOOD

Freezing homemade baby food is a great way to stay prepared and keep a variety of meals on hand. After preparing purée, let it cool to room temperature. To freeze it, divide the purée among clean, individual plastic ice cube trays with covers, being careful not to overfill the compartments. Once frozen, transfer the cubes to plastic bags, labeling each bag with the type of food and date prepared. Seal the bags tightly and return them to the freezer. (Freezer temperature should be 0°F [-18°C] or lower to prevent bacteria from forming.) Use the cubes within four to six weeks.

To serve, remove as many cubes as needed for each feeding, keeping in mind one cube is about 1 ounce (28 ml). You can defrost the cubes in the refrigerator, melt them over low heat in a small saucepan, stirring often, or defrost them in the microwave, covered with a microwave-safe lid or plate or parchment paper. (As noted earlier, do not use regular plastic wrap; the plastic may contain toxic substances that are released when heated.) Stir the purée well once defrosted, and let cool before serving.

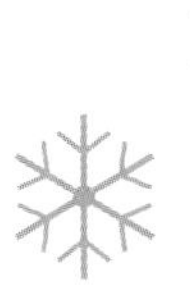

A Snowflake Means It's a Breeze to Freeze!

When you see a snowflake icon ❄ (this will be a repeating element on all noted recipes), this indicates a recipe is suitable for freezing. Fix and freeze these recipes whenever you have a free moment and save yourself loads of time in the long run!

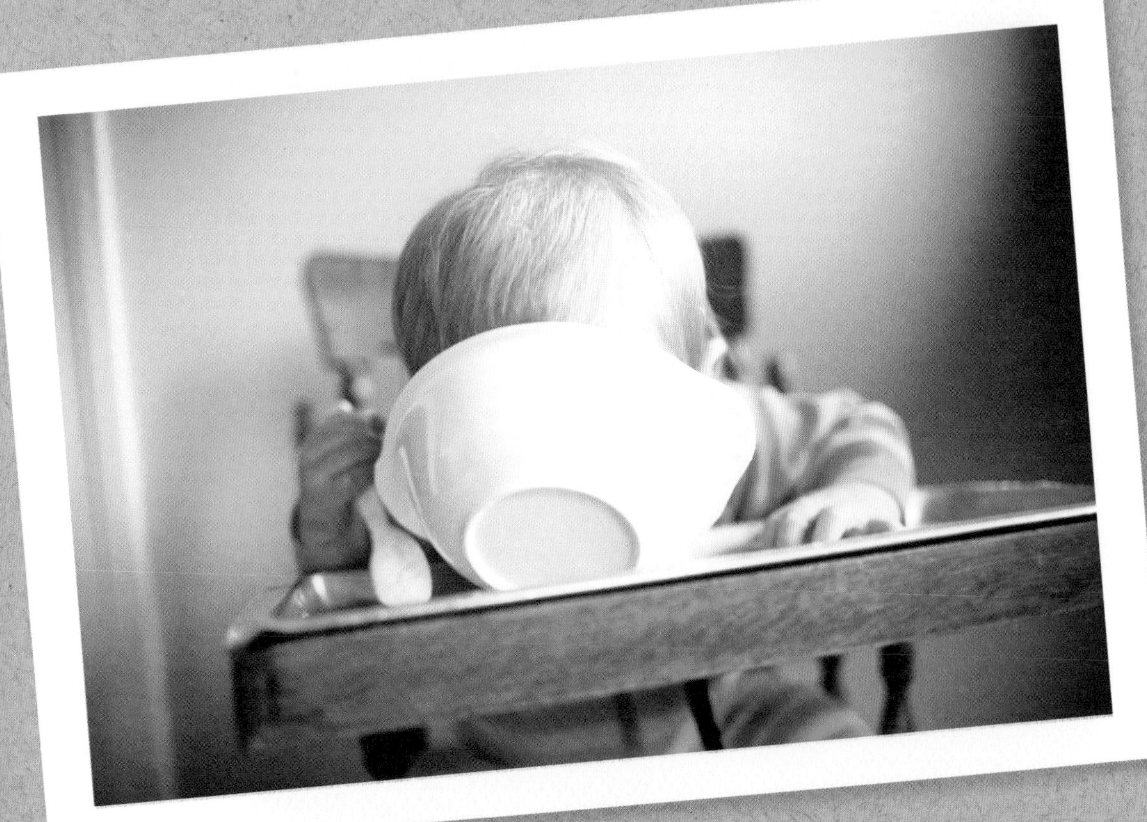

"A baby will make love stronger, days shorter, nights longer, bankroll smaller, home happier, clothes shabbier, the past forgotten, and the future worth living for."

— Author Unknown

CHAPTER TWO

Feeding Your Baby the Best—from Six to Eleven Months

Until your baby turns a year old, the majority of her nutrition will come from breast milk or formula. But at six months of age, it's time to start introducing her to solid food so that she can gradually develop a preference for different flavors and textures. In addition, by six months of age, your baby will have used up the iron stores she was born with, so she'll need to get this important mineral from food.

As your baby tries more and more foods, she'll eventually choose her favorites. The more variety in your little one's diet, the greater the probability her meals will contain all the nutrients she needs. Further, if your baby is used to eating many different foods, it will be easier to find several she likes and will accept if her appetite occasionally declines or becomes irregular.

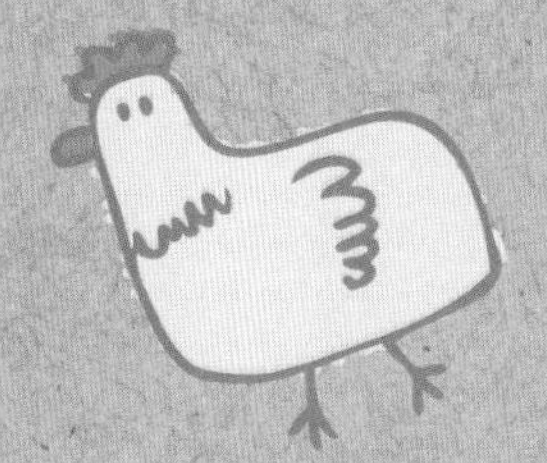

How Do I Know If My Baby Is Ready for Solid Food?

Each baby is unique, but around six months of age, most babies are ready to start solids and begin familiarizing themselves with spoon-feeding and the taste and texture of various foods.

Several physiological factors play a role in creating this need. The key factors at six months are as follows:

- Most of the iron supply a baby is born with has been used up; breast milk is not an adequate source of iron and it must be supplemented.
- Enzymes needed to digest solid food are now present.
- Infants are now able to swallow semi-solids without choking. (Babies are born with a strong sucking and extrusion reflex, which makes them instinctively push their tongue out. Until this reflex disappears, starting around four months of age, solids will automatically be pushed out of the mouth.)
- Up-and-down chewing ability begins.

Here are some signs to look for to determine whether your baby is ready for solid foods:

- Your baby consumes more than 32 ounces (950 ml) of breast milk or formula a day.
- Your baby's birth weight has doubled.
- Your baby can hold his neck steady and sit up with support.
- Your baby shows interest in food when others are eating.
- Your baby expresses a desire for food by leaning toward a spoon with an open mouth when hungry or leaning back and turning away when full.

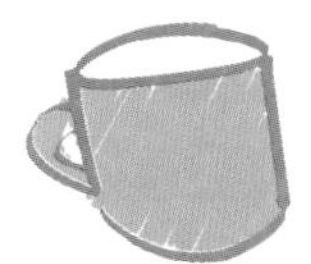

The Best Way to Introduce Solid Food

When your baby is ready, start by giving him baby cereal. Rice is a good choice because it's a single-grain infant cereal (meaning that only one grain is used), easy to digest, and least likely to cause intolerance or allergic reaction.

The best time to try any new food is in the morning after a partial breast- or bottle-feeding when your little one is not too hungry. If you give a new food in the evening, any potential reaction will probably occur during the night—and you likely do not want to be kept awake all night with a baby who is uncomfortable and unhappy. Once you know that there is no reaction to a new food, you can serve it at any time of day.

Before you give your baby her very first bite, test it on yourself to make sure it's tepid. Then fill a small weaning spoon with a little bit of cereal and gently put it on your baby's tongue. The first few times the cereal may wind up on her face or bib. Relax and enjoy this new experience; if you're relaxed, your baby will be as well. You're learning how to feed your baby, and your baby is learning how to eat. In a short time, you'll both have mastered it. Try one more spoonful and continue, unless she refuses, until the cereal is gone. This may seem like a tiny amount, but these initial feedings are mostly to get your baby used to new textures and tastes. The majority of her nourishment will still be obtained from breast milk or formula.

When rice cereal becomes well tolerated, you can gradually increase the amount to 2 to 4 tablespoons (28 to 55 g). These can be divided into two daily feedings. Remember, never force your baby to finish food that she refuses.

Where Should I Feed My Baby?

If your baby is able to sit up alone, use a highchair. Be sure to use the safety straps. If needed, place pillows on the sides for support. If your little one is still unsteady, sit him on your lap, head cradled in your arm, but in an upright position to prevent choking. Another alternative is to use an infant carrier, again in an upright position. Keep in mind, babies need to learn how to chew and swallow, so do not give semi-solids in a bottle.

Adding New Foods

If your infant refuses a new food, remove it and offer it again after a few days. Babies who are coaxed or forced to eat a new food may learn to dislike it. After retrying foods with no pressure, infants will often accept food they initially rejected.

CEREALS

After three or four days of accepting rice cereal, introduce another single-grain cereal, such as barley or oatmeal. Use the same rule every time you introduce a new food: Serve it for three to four days and watch carefully for any signs of intolerance or allergy before trying another.

JUICE

After you've introduced a variety of cereals, try some fruit juices. Start with apple, white grape, or pear juice. (At this age, it's best to use commercial baby juice, since you won't be able to pasteurize homemade juice. Pasteurization helps kill bacteria that can cause food poisoning.)

Dilute the juice by half with water and offer it in a small cup with a covered lid and drinking spout. Never put juice in a baby bottle. Juice is a sugary breeding ground for germs, and when babies continuously suck on the bottle or are put to sleep with a bottle of juice, tooth decay and even ear infections can result. In addition, according to the American Academy of Pediatrics, feeding babies juice in a bottle can contribute to over-nutrition and precipitate obesity. If it's sucking that your baby finds soothing, try a pacifier instead of a bottle.

To begin, start with 1 ounce (28 ml) and gradually work up to 4 ounces (120 ml) of diluted juice until your baby is eight months old. After eight months, it is optional to dilute juices, but don't serve more than a ½ cup (120 ml) a day. Too much juice can spoil your baby's appetite and cause cramping and diarrhea.

FRUITS AND VEGGIES

Once your baby is comfortable with cereals, try other new foods. Start with fruits or vegetables or, better still, alternate between the two. Use fruits and vegetables rich in vitamin C, such as pears and sweet potatoes. They should be cooked, peeled, and puréed. Use the same method for introducing fruits and vegetables as you did with cereals. Start with 1 tablespoon (15 g) per serving. After a day or two, if there is no sign of intolerance or allergy, add another tablespoon. Gradually increase the amount to 2 to 4 tablespoons (28 to 55 g) twice daily (¼ to ½ cup [55 to 115 g] a day total), depending on your baby's appetite.

INTRODUCING SOLIDS: BABY'S MONTH-BY-MONTH GUIDE

Use this handy chart to identify what foods your baby can start eating each month.

FOOD	SIX MONTHS	SEVEN MONTHS	EIGHT MONTHS	NINE MONTHS	TEN MONTHS	ELEVEN MONTHS
BABY CEREAL	single-grain rice, barley, oatmeal		single-grain wheat			rice, cream of wheat, oatmeal, barley, multigrain
JUICE	dilute half-and-half with water: apple, pear, white grape	dilute half-and-half with water: peach, nectarine, prune	dilute half-and-half with water: apricot, blueberry, carrot	dilute with water (optional): red grape, cantaloupe, papaya nectar	dilute with water (optional): cherry, kiwi	dilute with water (optional): cranberry, pineapple, raspberry
VEGETABLES (cooked)	sweet potatoes, peas	squash (acorn, butternut, yellow), potatoes, zucchini	carrots, string beans, wax beans	broccoli, cauliflower, spinach	cabbage, parsnip, leek, bell peppers, parsley, celery	brussels sprouts, turnips, rutabaga, beets, kale, Romaine lettuce (raw)
FRUITS *very ripe	apples, pears, avocadoes*, bananas*	nectar-ines, peaches, plums, prunes	apricots*; dried, cooked apricots; blueberries; seedless watermelon	cantaloupe, papaya	kiwi, melon, cherry halves	pineapple, raisins (soft or cooked), grape halves, figs, raspberries
DAIRY, (whole fat)			cottage cheese	yogurt	cream cheese, mascarpone, fresh or soft mozzarella, Jack, Swiss	ricotta, Cheddar, goat, Parmesan, Romano
MISCELLANEOUS			hard-cooked egg yolk, rice, rice noodles, barley, baby crackers, plain oat Cheerios	chicken, beef, ham, tofu	pancakes, waffles, legumes (lentils and split peas)	polenta, couscous, legumes (beans: black, white, red, lima, or refried)

PLEASING PURÉES FOR YOUR LITTLE PEA:

RECIPES FOR SIX MONTHS

While every baby is different, most enjoy the first foods they're given. Keep in mind, their first "meals" will really be tiny tastes of this and that. They'll let you know what they like and what they don't, so look for their little cues. And once they have a selection of favorite purées and cereals, feel free to experiment, blending different recipes together for even more variety.

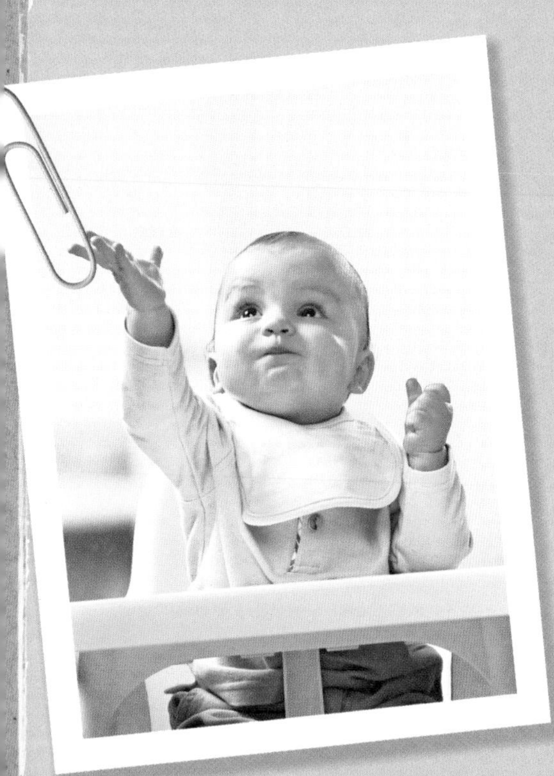

Iron-Clad Your Baby's Diet

Iron deficiency is common among babies and toddlers and occurs because they often "grow out" of the amount of iron they're born with. While breast milk is thought to contain all the iron a baby needs, once an infant is weaned, it is important to ensure that he is eating enough iron-rich foods to compensate for the reduced iron intake from breast milk. Important sources of iron for infants include iron-fortified infant formula and cereals, dark green vegetables, legumes, avocados, brown rice (another great reason to make your own cereal), cooked egg yolks and meat. Also, feeding your baby foods that are high in vitamin C alongside iron-rich foods aids the absorption of iron, so try pairing the foods that follow with vitamin-C rich foods like papaya and cauliflower.

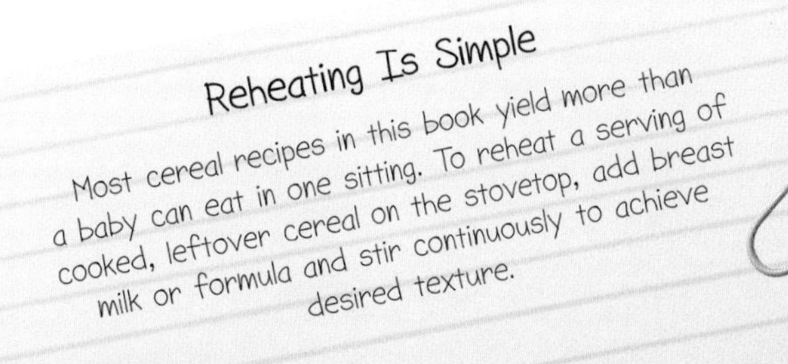

Reheating Is Simple

Most cereal recipes in this book yield more than a baby can eat in one sitting. To reheat a serving of cooked, leftover cereal on the stovetop, add breast milk or formula and stir continuously to achieve desired texture.

Mighty Mouthful Rice Cereal

White rice is considered a refined grain having little nutrition. Brown rice is a much healthier choice, since it contains important B vitamins, fiber, iron and essential fatty acids.

1/2 cup (120 ml) water

1/4 cup (40 g) ground brown rice

1/4 cup (60 ml) breast milk or formula

STOVETOP METHOD: Bring water to boil in saucepan. Add the ground brown rice while stirring constantly. Simmer for 10 minutes, continuing to whisk. Allow mixture to cool slightly and then transfer purée to blender. Whirl until smooth, adding breast milk or formula to achieve desired consistency. Let cool and serve at room temperature.

YIELD: 8 baby servings, 2 tablespoons (28 g) each

EACH SERVING (if using breast milk) CONTAINS: 28.4 calories; 0.5 g total fat; 0.2 grams saturated fat; 1.4 mg cholesterol; 1.6 mg sodium; 5.1 g carbohydrates; 0.2 g dietary fiber; 0.52 g protein; 4.4 mg calcium; 0.1 mg iron; 16.3 IU vitamin A; and 0.4 mg vitamin C.

Baby's First Oatmeal

Oats are a good source of many nutrients, including vitamin E, zinc, iron, and protein.

3/4 cup (175 ml) water

1/4 cup (20 g) ground old-fashioned rolled oatmeal

1/4 cup (60 ml) breast milk or formula

STOVETOP METHOD: Bring water to boil in saucepan. Add the ground oatmeal while stirring constantly. Simmer for 10 minutes, whisking constantly. Mix in formula or breast milk. Let cool and serve at room temperature.

YIELD: 4 baby servings, 2 tablespoons (28 g) each

EACH SERVING (if using breast milk) CONTAINS: 34.7 calories; 1.1 g total fat; 0.4 grams saturated fat; 2.2 mg cholesterol; 3.3 mg sodium; 5.3 g carbohydrates; 0.7 g dietary fiber; 1 g protein; 8.6 mg calcium; 0.3 mg iron; 32.7 IU vitamin A; and 0.78 mg vitamin C.

Make Your Own Baby Cereal in Two Easy Steps!

Baby cereal, a staple in these beginning months, is easy to make, especially when you have the ingredients already prepared. To do this, pulverize in a basic blender three to four cups each of brown rice, oats, and barley. The consistency of the grains should be like powder. Then, store each powder separately in containers with tight-fitting lids. (Sugar and flour canisters work well for this purpose.) When you're ready to make cereal, all you'll have to do is scoop out what you need and begin cooking.

Perfect Apple Purée ❄

Fuji, Gala, or Golden Delicious apples are all good choices for this purée. They are naturally sweet, not tart, and will provide the best results.

1 sweet, ripe apple

¼ to ⅓ cup (60 to 80 ml) water (if cooking on stovetop)

MICROWAVE METHOD: Wash, quarter, and core but do not peel the apple. Place the apple on a plate, cut sides down. Microwave on high, uncovered, 3 to 4 minutes until the apple is soft. Let the apple cool and then peel. Purée in a blender for 30 seconds or until the apple is completely smooth.

STOVETOP METHOD: Wash, peel, quarter, and core the apple and cut into small pieces. Add water to a small saucepan and bring to a boil. Add the apple pieces to the boiling water, cover, reduce the heat, and simmer 10 minutes or until the apple is soft. Check occasionally to see if you need to add more water. Allow mixture to cool slightly and then whirl the apple and water in a blender 1 to 2 minutes until the apple is completely puréed. If needed, add 1 to 2 tablespoons (15 to 28 ml) more water.

This recipe, covered tightly, will last for 2 days in the refrigerator.

YIELD: 3 baby servings, 2 heaping tablespoons (30 to 40 g) each

EACH SERVING CONTAINS: 25.9 calories; 0.1 g total fat; 0.0 grams saturated fat; 0.0 mg cholesterol; 0.5 mg sodium; 6.9 g carbohydrates; 1.2 g dietary fiber; 0.1 g protein; 3.0 mg calcium; 0.1 mg iron; 26.8 IU vitamin A; and 2.3 mg vitamin C.

Sweet Pear Purée ❄

This recipe tastes best using Bartlett, Anjou, or Bosc pears since they're sweet, juicy, and provide a nice texture. Pears are a good source of vitamin C, potassium, and fiber.

1 sweet, ripe pear

¼ to ⅓ cup (60 to 80 ml) water (if cooking on stovetop)

MICROWAVE METHOD: Wash, peel, quarter, and core the pear. Place it on a plate and microwave on high 5 minutes or until soft. Allow mixture to cool slightly and then whirl in a blender for 30 seconds or until the pear is completely puréed.

STOVETOP METHOD: Wash, peel, quarter, and core the pear and cut into small pieces. Add the water to a small saucepan and bring to a boil. Add the pear pieces to the boiling water, cover, reduce heat, and simmer 10 minutes, or until the pear is soft. Check occasionally to see if you need to add more water. Allow mixture to cool slightly and then whirl in a blender for 30 seconds or until the pear is completely puréed.

This recipe, covered tightly, will last for 2 days in the refrigerator.

YIELD: 3 baby servings, 2 heaping tablespoons (30 to 40 g) each

EACH SERVING CONTAINS: 34.4 calories; 0.1 g total fat; 0.0 grams saturated fat; 0.0 mg cholesterol; 0.6 mg sodium; 9.2 g carbohydrates; 1.8 g dietary fiber; 0.2 g protein; 5.3 mg calcium; 0.1 mg iron; 13.7 IU vitamin A; and 2.5 mg vitamin C.

Best Banana Sauté ❄

Bananas are bursting with nutrients. They're an ideal fruit to choose for one of your baby's first "solid" meals.

1/3 very ripe banana

1 teaspoon butter

STOVETOP METHOD: Cut banana into pieces and sauté in butter for 2 minutes. Mash with fork. Add breast milk or formula if too thick.

This recipe, covered tightly, will last for 2 days in the refrigerator.

YIELD: 3 baby servings, 1 tablespoon (15 g) each

EACH SERVING CONTAINS: 22.8 calories; 1.3 g total fat; 0.9 grams saturated fat; 3.3 mg cholesterol; 0.1 mg sodium; 3.0 g carbohydrates; 0.3 g dietary fiber; 0.1 g protein; 0.7 mg calcium; 0.0 mg iron; 52.8 IU vitamin A; and 1.1 mg vitamin C.

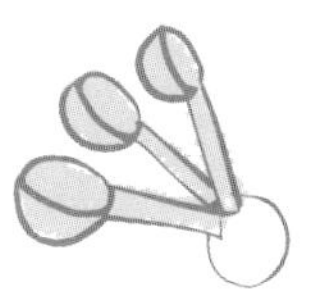

Ready, Set, Go Avocado Purée

Make no-cook purées just before your baby is ready to eat them. Their texture and color is best when fresh. (This is especially true with avocado, which browns quickly due to oxidation.)

1/2 small ripe avocado

Peel and pit avocado. Scoop out flesh and mash with the back of a spoon. Add a tablespoon (15 ml) of breast milk or formula if the consistency is too thick.

YIELD: 4 baby servings, 1 tablespoon (15 g) each

EACH SERVING CONTAINS: 25.1 calories; 3.7 g total fat; 0.5 grams saturated fat; 0.0 mg cholesterol; 1.8 mg sodium; 2.1 g carbohydrates; 1.7 g dietary fiber; 0.5 g protein; 3.0 mg calcium; 0.1 mg iron; 36.7 IU vitamin A; and 2.5 mg vitamin C.

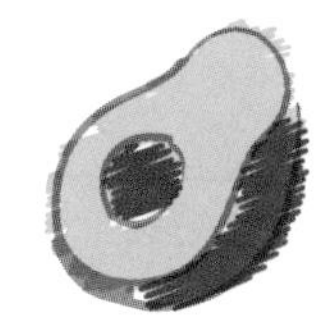

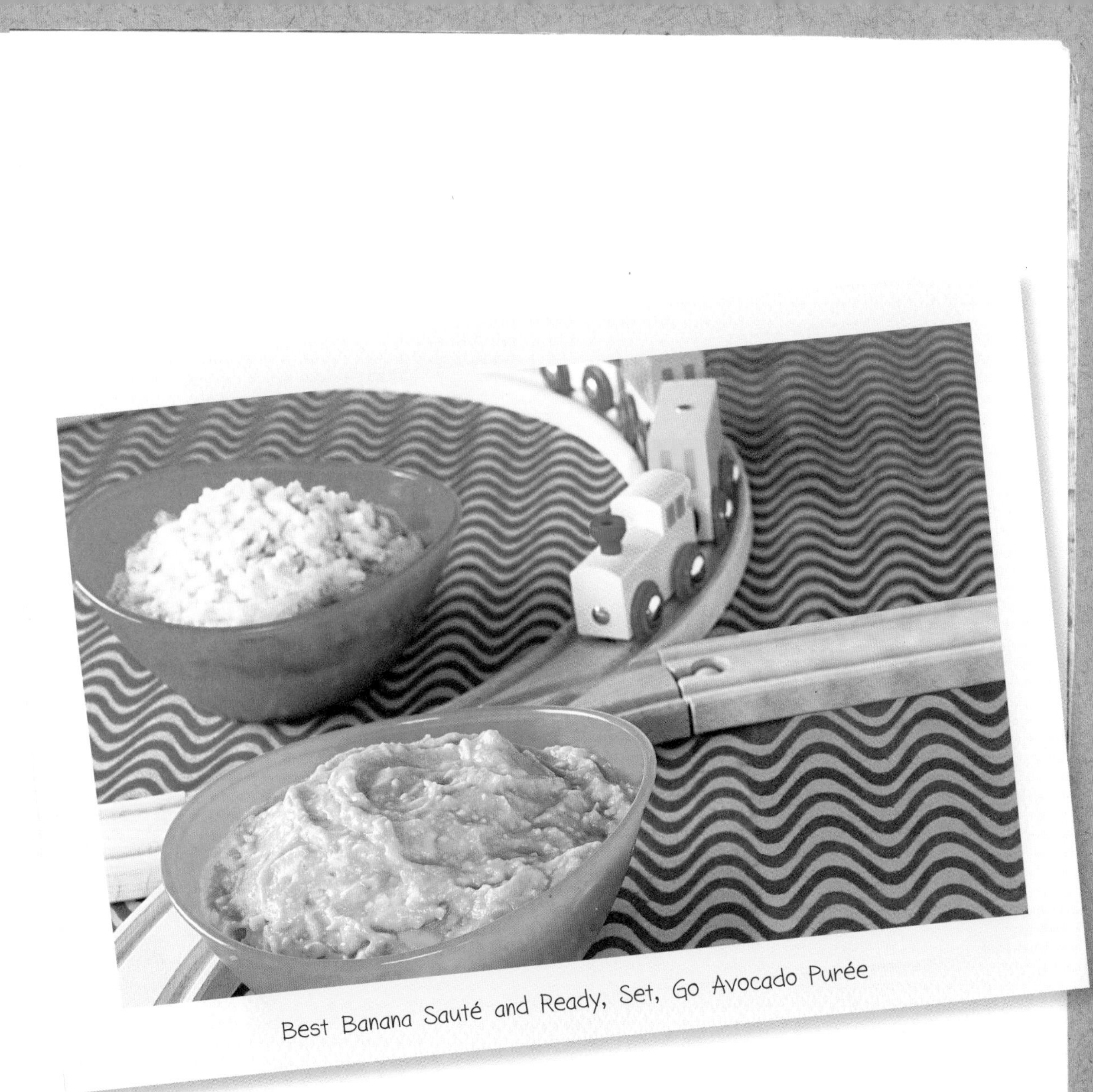

Best Banana Sauté and Ready, Set, Go Avocado Purée

Double Whammy Banan-y

Combine banana and avocado for a new flavor combination. If you're unsure your baby will enjoy this combination (say she doesn't prefer one or the other of these two fruits), mash them separately and alternate feeding a spoon of avocado and a spoon of banana.

2 tablespoons (28 g) mashed avocado

¼ ripe mashed banana

In a bowl, mix together the avocado and banana.

YIELD: 4 baby servings, 1 tablespoon (15 g) each

EACH SERVING CONTAINS: 14.6 calories; 1.1 g total fat; 0.2 grams saturated fat; 0.0 mg cholesterol; 0.6 mg sodium; 2.3 g carbohydrates; 0.7 g dietary fiber; 0.2 g protein; 1.2 mg calcium; 0.1 mg iron; 15.2 IU vitamin A; and 1.4 mg vitamin C.

Perfectly Paired Fruit and Grain Oatmeal

Oatmeal's mild flavor goes very well with fruits such as apple, banana, and pear. Always make oats with breast milk or formula since they contribute much-needed calcium and protein to the diet.

¼ cup (20 g) ground old-fashioned rolled oatmeal

½ cup (120 ml) breast milk or formula

⅓ ripe banana

STOVETOP METHOD: Combine ground oatmeal and breast milk or formula. Bring to a boil. Simmer for 5 minutes, stirring occasionally until liquid is mostly absorbed. Remove from heat and cover; let stand for 5 minutes. Mash banana and add to the cooked cereal. Thin with additional breast milk or formula as necessary.

YIELD: 4 baby servings, 2 tablespoons (28 g) each

EACH SERVING (if using breast milk) CONTAINS: 54.2 calories; 1.8 g total fat; 0.7 grams saturated fat; 4.3 mg cholesterol; 5.6 mg sodium; 8.6 g carbohydrates; 0.9 g dietary fiber; 1.2 g protein; 13.6 mg calcium; 0.3 mg iron; 71.6 IU vitamin A; and 2.4 mg vitamin C.

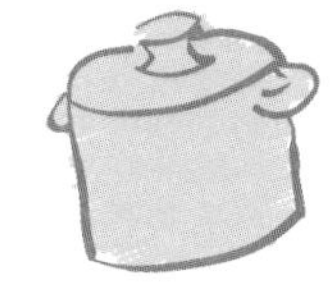

A Potato with High-Chair Creds

Sweet potatoes are one of the most nutritious vegetables you can feed your baby because they contain beta-carotene, a naturally occurring pigment found in yellow, orange, and red fruits and vegetables. Beta-carotene is converted by the body to vitamin A, which is important for good vision, healthy skin, normal growth, and protection from infections.

From birth to six months of age, babies get their required beta-carotene from breast milk and some formula brands. For infants six months to one year, 500 mcg of beta carotene each day is sufficient, or the equivalent of 2 tablespoons (28 g) of sweet potato purée.

Kiss the Cook Pear-Potato Purée ❄

Adding pear to sweet potato creates a pleasing, sweet/savory flavor combination. If your baby isn't fond of sweet potatoes, adding a touch of pear purée just might do the trick.

1 tablespoon (15 g) Oh So Sweet Potato Purée (page 34)

1 tablespoon (15 g) Sweet Pear Purée (page 29)

Combine the two purées and serve warm or chilled.

YIELD: 1 baby serving, or 2 tablespoons (28 g)

EACH SERVING CONTAINS: 32.7 calories; 0.2 g total fat; 0.2 grams saturated fat; 1.4 mg cholesterol; 7.9 mg sodium; 7.2 g carbohydrates; 1.2 g dietary fiber; 0.4 g protein; 7.7 mg calcium; 0.1 mg iron; 528.7 IU vitamin A; and 3.3 mg vitamin C.

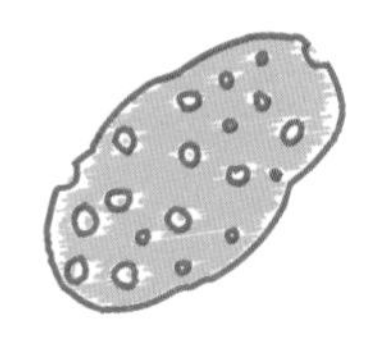

Potassium-Powered Potato-Banana Purée ❄

Cooked sweet potatoes can be stored in the refrigerator for up to a week, and they can also be frozen. Make a few batches of this recipe to have on hand for later; it's just a matter of combining equal portions of each ingredient, so it should be a breeze.

1 tablespoon (15 g) Oh So Sweet Potato Purée (page 34)

1 tablespoon (15 g) mashed banana

Mix together the sweet potato and banana. You may want to serve this dish with a little breast milk or formula on the side.

YIELD: 1 baby serving, or 2 tablespoons (28 g)

EACH SERVING CONTAINS: 28.0 calories; 0.6 g total fat; 0.4 grams saturated fat; 1.4 mg cholesterol; 7.7 mg sodium; 5.8 g carbohydrates; 0.7 g dietary fiber; 0.5 g protein; 5.7 mg calcium; 0.4 mg iron; 530.8 IU vitamin A; and 3.2 mg vitamin C.

Yummy Recipe Variation

Use puréed apple or puréed pear instead of the banana for a yummy variation of this recipe.

Oh So Sweet Potato Purée ❄

If using the oven method, lightly grease the skin of the sweet potato with butter before baking—it will peel more easily once cooled. Do not wrap the potato in aluminum foil, however, because it will steam and lose its sweet, syrupy flavor.

1 sweet potato

½ to 1 cup (120 to 235 ml) water, apple juice, pear juice, breast milk, or formula

Unsalted butter (if baking)

MICROWAVE METHOD: Wash and scrub the sweet potato. Prick the skin of the potato with a fork in several places. Microwave on high 8 to 10 minutes or until the potato is soft. Let the potato cool until it's easy to handle and peel. Cut the potato into chunks. Place in a blender with ½ cup (120 ml) liquid and purée until completely smooth. Add up to ½ cup (120 ml) additional liquid if needed. Serve lukewarm.

OVEN METHOD: Preheat the oven to 400°F (200°C, gas mark 6). Wash and scrub the sweet potato. Rub the potato with a little butter and place on a baking sheet. Bake until soft, 30 to 50 minutes, depending on size. Cool, peel, and chop into chunks. Place in a blender with ½ cup (120 ml) liquid and purée until completely smooth. Add another ½ cup (120 ml) liquid if needed.

This recipe, covered tightly, will last for 2 days in the refrigerator.

YIELD: 3 baby servings, ¼ cup (55 g) each

EACH SERVING (if using breast milk) CONTAINS: 62.1 calories; 1.8 g total fat; 0.8 grams saturated fat; 5.6 mg cholesterol; 30.3 mg sodium; 10.5 g carbohydrates; 1.3 g dietary fiber; 1.1 g protein; 19.8 mg calcium; 0.3 mg iron; 2087.1 IU vitamin A; and 8.1 mg vitamin C.

Baby's Favorite Barley Cereal

Barley is a versatile cereal grain with a nut-like taste. It's a good source of vitamin A, folate, and even protein. It also goes great served with any fruit or vegetable purée.

1 cup (235 ml) water

¼ cup (46 g) ground quick-cook barley

STOVETOP METHOD: Bring water to a boil in saucepan. Add the barley and simmer for 10 minutes, whisking constantly. Mix in formula or breast milk if needed to achieve desired consistency and add puréed fruit or vegetables for variety, if you wish. Serve lukewarm.

YIELD: 4 baby servings, 2 tablespoons (28 g) each

EACH SERVING CONTAINS: 71.6 calories; 0.3 g total fat; 0.0 grams saturated fat; 0.0 mg cholesterol; 1.6 mg sodium; 9.8 g carbohydrates; 2.0 g dietary fiber; 1.3 g protein; 3.1 mg calcium; 0.3 mg iron; 0.0 IU vitamin A; and 0.0 mg vitamin C.

Yummy Recipe Variation

You can enhance the flavor of this recipe by adding mashed banana or other leftover purée.

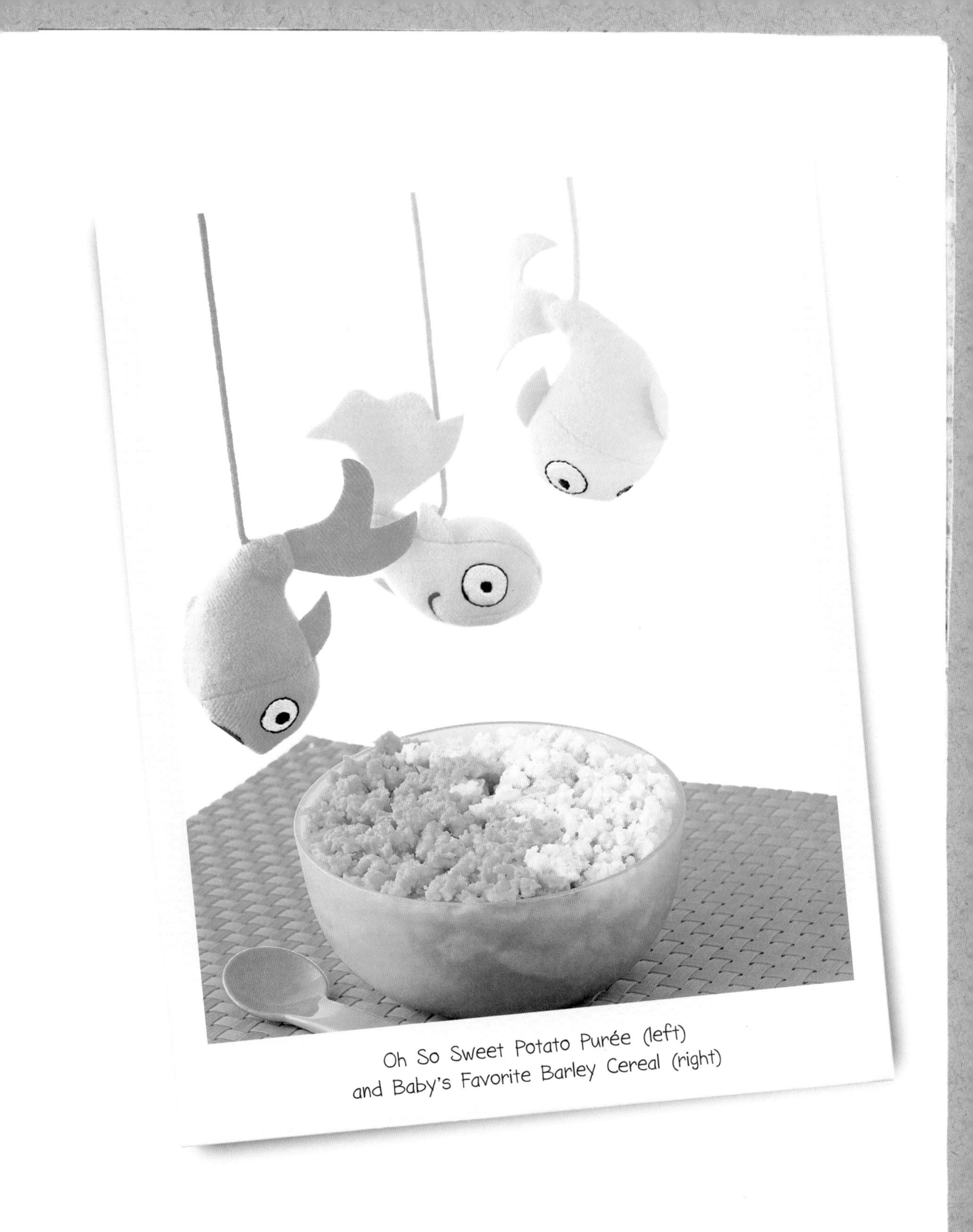

Oh So Sweet Potato Purée (left)
and Baby's Favorite Barley Cereal (right)

Apple-a-Day Oatmeal

If your baby is hungry or if you don't have ground oats on hand, mix homemade apple purée with iron-fortified baby oats for a nourishing meal in minutes. This is another recipe that can be easily multiplied for a larger amount; the 1:1 ratio stays the same.

1 tablespoon (15 g) Baby's First Oatmeal (page 28), or whole grain baby oatmeal prepared with breast milk or formula

1 tablespoon (15 g) Perfect Apple Purée (page 29)

Mix the two ingredients together and serve.

YIELD: 1 baby serving, or 2 tablespoons (28 g)

EACH SERVING CONTAINS: 30.1 calories; 0.9 g total fat; 0.3 grams saturated fat; 2.2 mg cholesterol; 2.6 mg sodium; 5.0 g carbohydrates; 0.5 g dietary fiber; 0.8 g protein; 42.9 mg calcium; 5.0 mg iron; 37.2 IU vitamin A; and 1.2 mg vitamin C.

What Is a Seckel Pear?

Seckel pears, also known as sugar pears, are delicious, miniature-sized pears. They're in season between August and January. Given their size, they're ideal for making baby food purées.

Yummy Apple-Pear Purée ❄

Pears are a rich source of nutrients and a good source of vitamin C, and they're always available at the grocery store. Did you know that there are more than 3,000 varieties of pears?

1 ripe Seckel pear or ½ pear of another variety

¼ cup (60 g) unsweetened applesauce

¼ cup (60 ml) pear nectar or unsweetened apple juice

STOVETOP METHOD: Peel, core, and chop the pear. Put it into a small saucepan with the applesauce and cook covered on medium heat for 5 to 7 minutes until mixture is soft. Allow mixture to cool slightly and then add to blender with pear nectar and whip into a smooth purée.

This recipe, covered tightly, will last for 2 days in the refrigerator.

YIELD: 4 baby servings, 2 tablespoons (28 g) each

EACH SERVING (if using pear nectar) CONTAINS: 28.4 calories; 0.0 g total fat; 0.0 grams saturated fat; 0.0 mg cholesterol; 1.0 mg sodium; 7.4 g carbohydrates; 0.9 g dietary fiber; 0.1 g protein; 6.1 mg calcium; 0.1 mg iron; 9.5 IU vitamin A; and 3.7 mg vitamin C.

A Dozen Helpful Hints for Introducing Baby to Purées

1. Never give food while your baby is lying down, crying, or laughing.
2. Always test food first for appropriate temperature.
3. Don't add salt, spices, or sweeteners to any foods or juices during the first twelve months.
4. Don't give excessive amounts of juice. This may decrease your baby's desire for nursing or formula, which is still the most important food source, and too much juice can cause diarrhea.
5. Try only one new food at a time. When introducing a new food, serve it for three or four days, watching carefully for any reaction before moving on to another new food.
6. Be aware that there may be changes in your baby's bowel movements once he starts eating solids. This is normal. Also, a breast-fed baby will probably have more frequent stools, while there may be no change with a bottle-fed baby. Keep in mind that most fruits, especially prunes, have a mild laxative effect, which is also helpful to know if your baby is constipated.
7. If your baby opens his mouth, he may be asking for food. When he shuts his mouth, spits food out, or turns his head away, it probably means he does not like the food or he is full.
8. Never force your baby to eat. Remove the food and offer it again when he indicates he is hungry and ready to eat.
9. Allow infants to eat at their own pace, and be very patient. For babies, every bite is a new adventure.
10. If your baby rejects a new food, wait a few days and try again. Again, be patient; it may take several attempts to be successful. If you don't force the food, your baby may eventually accept it without any fuss.
11. Do not dilute cereal and feed it from a bottle; this can cause tooth decay.
12. Avoid using teething pain relief medicine before mealtimes, as it may make chewing difficult.

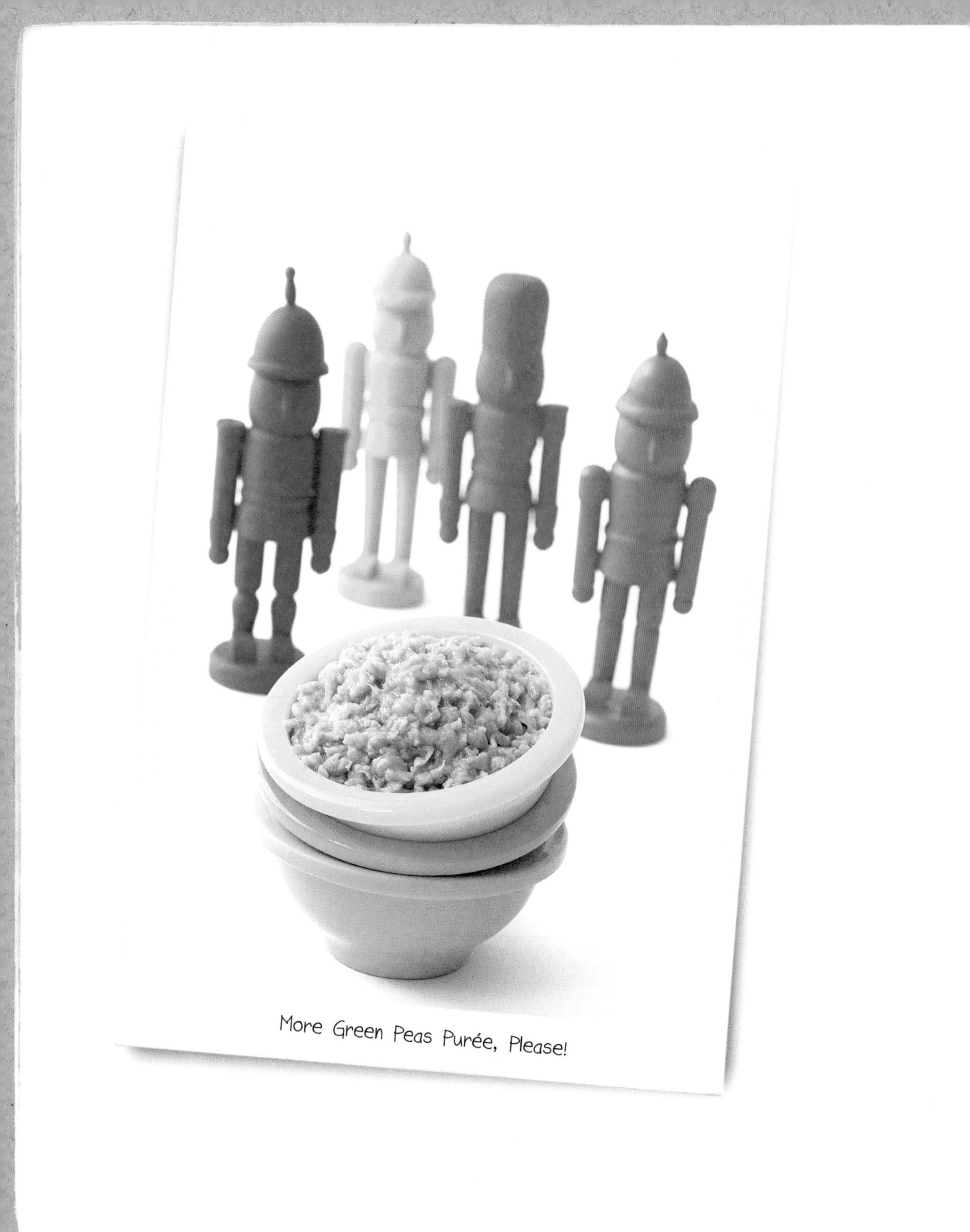

More Green Peas Purée, Please!

More Green Peas Purée, Please! ❄

Until your baby is used to the flavor of peas, you may want to add breast milk or formula to mellow the taste. To freeze, double the recipe, and follow the directions for freezing purées (page 19).

1 cup (160 g) fresh or frozen peas

¼ cup (60 ml) water

¼ cup (60 ml) breast milk or formula

MICROWAVE METHOD: Place the peas and water in a glass dish. Cover and microwave on high for 5 minutes, until the peas are soft. Allow to cool slightly and then place the peas in a blender with the breast milk or formula and purée 1 minute, until smooth. Adjust the amount of liquid depending on how thin you want the purée.

STOVETOP METHOD: Bring the water to a boil in a small pan. Add the peas and return to a boil. Cover, reduce heat to low, and simmer 5 to 6 minutes, until the peas are tender. Stir once during cooking. Allow to cool slightly and then place the peas and water in a blender. Add the breast milk or formula and purée 1 minute, until smooth.

YIELD: 3 baby servings, 2 tablespoons (28 g) each

EACH SERVING CONTAINS: 83.6 calories; 0.9 g total fat; 0.4 grams saturated fat; 2.9 mg cholesterol; 3.5 mg sodium; 7.4 g carbohydrates; 2.0 g dietary fiber; 2.2 g protein; 7.2 mg calcium; 0.5 mg iron; 242.5 IU vitamin A; and 4.0 mg vitamin C.

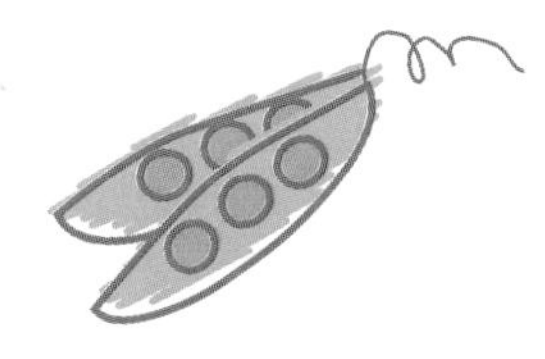

Not All Peas Are Created Equal

Peas cooked in the microwave contain twice as much vitamin C as commercially prepared baby food peas.

HEALTHY NEW TASTES TO ENTICE AND EXPLORE:

RECIPES FOR SEVEN MONTHS

At seven months, the bulk of your baby's nourishment will still come from breast milk or formula (typically from five daily feedings, or 26 to 32 ounces [765 to 950 ml] total), but she will also be progressing in her development of the up-and-down chewing motion. With this in mind, continue to offer recipes in the six months section, but begin progressing from a purée to a soft, mashed texture. Let your baby explore this new change with ease—she's certain to warm up to it in no time.

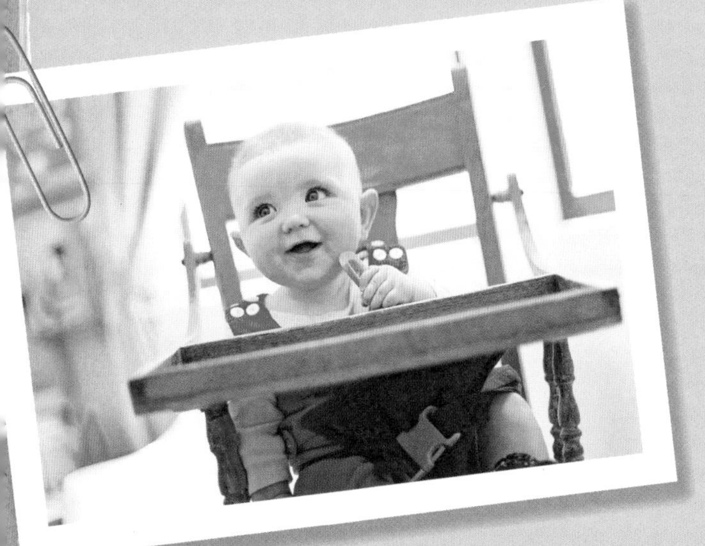

Helpful Hints for the High Chair

Following are some reminders and recommendations for preparing food for your seven-month-old:

- Wash, peel, seed, cut, and cook all vegetables. Summer squash, such as zucchini and yellow crookneck, are the exception to this rule; they do not need to be peeled (but everything else applies).
- Wash, peel, core, cut, and cook apples and then mash. Pears, if very ripe, can be washed, peeled, cored, and cut and then mashed well with a fork (without cooking). Fresh, ripe peaches, plums, and nectarines can also be washed, peeled, pitted, and puréed without cooking.
- Dilute juice by half with water. Give no more than a ½ cup (120 ml) diluted juice a day (¼ cup [60 ml] juice + ¼ cup [60 ml) water].

And when it comes time to feeding your little one, remember the following:

- Both food and drink should be served lukewarm or at room temperature.
- You should continue to introduce new foods one at a time every three days or so and watch for reactions. See "Understanding Allergies and Food Intolerance: How to Know the Difference," page 209.
- You should continue feeding single-grain cereal to your baby, eventually working up to ¼ cup (55 g) and then ½ cup (115 g), which can be divided into two ¼-cup (55 g) feedings a day. Serve with juice or fruits rich in vitamin C.

NEW BITES FOR YOUR SEVEN-MONTH-OLD

At seven months, you can make these additions to your baby's diet:

VEGETABLES (cooked)	• Acorn squash • Butternut squash • Potatoes • Yellow squash • Pumpkin • Zucchini
FRUITS	• Nectarines • Peaches • Plums • Prunes
JUICE (diluted with water)	• Peach • Nectarine • Prune

The Appestat: Your Baby's True Hunger Indicator

Recent research shows that infants are born with an instinct, referred to as their *appestat,* that sends a "stop eating" signal to the part of the brain that controls appetite. Trusting this inborn knowledge of how much food will satisfy your baby's appetite lays the foundation for good eating habits.To heed your baby's appestat, pay close attention to when he signals that he is full—and be equally attentive when he signals that he is hungry. Here are clues that your child's appestat has told him that he's had enough:

NEWBORN	• Spits out nipple or falls asleep
SIX TO TWELVE MONTHS	• Turns head away to regulate pace or end feeding • Refuses to open mouth • Spits out food • Stores food in mouth • Pushes dish, cup, or bottle away
ONE TO TWO YEARS	• Shakes head no • Puts hand over mouth • Pushes away the hand that offers food • Uses simple words like "No," "Don't," or "Away" • Pushes away or throws plate, cup, or spoon
TWO TO THREE YEARS	• Combines words, such as "All done" or "Get down" • Pushes away plate • Tries to remove bib

Infants and toddlers who follow their hunger and satiety cues, eating only as much as their bodies need for good health, develop habits of moderation that should last a lifetime.

However, as important as it is to let your child judge how much food she wants, it can be one of the most difficult things for a parent to do. Many parents tend to give infants and toddlers larger portions than necessary—and then expect them to finish all the food on their plates. If a child's natural appestat breaks down because she is frequently encouraged to eat when she is full, feeding problems can develop, and determining when and how much to eat may become a battle between parent and child. To keep this from happening, always start with small portions, and then let your little one tell you in her own way if she wants more.

Zoom Zoom Zucchini ❄

Zucchini are part of the squash family. They contribute folate, vitamin C, and potassium to the diet.

1 small zucchini

¼ cup (60 ml) water

STOVETOP METHOD: Wash and trim the ends of the zucchini. Cut in half lengthwise and slice each half into ½-inch (12 mm) pieces. Place zucchini in a small pan with water. Cover and bring to a boil. Reduce the heat and simmer 5 minutes. Allow mixture to cool slightly and then transfer the zucchini and water to a blender and purée.

This recipe, covered tightly, will last for 2 days in the refrigerator.

YIELD: 5 baby servings, 2 tablespoons (28 g) each

EACH SERVING CONTAINS: 9.5 calories; 0.2 g total fat; 0.0 grams saturated fat; 0.0 mg cholesterol; 1.4 mg sodium; 1.4 g carbohydrates; 0.5 g dietary fiber; 1.2 g protein; 9.5 mg calcium; 0.4 mg iron; 220.5 IU vitamin A; and mg 15.3 vitamin C.

Sunrise Squash Purée ❄

Squash are very high in vitamins A and C. Yellow squash have a bumpy, yellow skin and taste best when they're about 6 inches (15 cm) in length.

1 small yellow squash

1 tablespoon (15 ml) apple juice or water (if microwaving)

⅓ cup (80 ml) water (if cooking on stovetop)

MICROWAVE METHOD: Wash and trim the ends of the squash. Cut in half lengthwise and slice each half into ½-inch (12 mm) pieces. Place squash in a microwave-safe dish, cover, and microwave on high 3 minutes. Add apple juice and mash with a fork or place the squash and apple juice in a blender and purée.

STOVETOP METHOD: Wash and trim the ends of the squash. Cut in half lengthwise and slice each half into ½ inch (12 mm) pieces. Place the squash in a small pan with ⅓ cup (80 ml) water. Cover and simmer 5 minutes or until the squash is soft. Allow squash to cool slightly and then place in a blender with 1 tablespoon (15 ml) of the cooking water and purée. Add more liquid if needed.

This recipe, covered tightly, will last for 2 days in the refrigerator.

YIELD: 2 baby servings, 2 tablespoons (28 g) each

EACH SERVING (if using apple juice) CONTAINS: 64.7 calories; 0.1 g total fat; 0.0 grams saturated fat; 0.0 mg cholesterol; 1.5 mg sodium; 2.7 g carbohydrates; 0.6 g dietary fiber; 0.7 g protein; 12.3 mg calcium; 0.2 mg iron; 113.4 IU vitamin A; and 11.8 mg vitamin C.

Creamy Butternut Squash Purée ❄

When first introducing this squash to your baby, mix it with a little breast milk or formula. After, you can try mixing it with Perfect Apple Purée (page 29) or Naturally Sweet Apricot Purée (page 56) for variety.

½ small butternut squash

2 tablespoons (28 ml) water

MICROWAVE METHOD: Seed and peel squash and cut in half lengthwise. Place in a microwave-safe dish, add water, and cover. Microwave on high 8 to 10 minutes, until soft. Allow mixture to cool slightly and then purée in a blender 30 seconds. Add a little breast milk or formula if wanted to achieve the desired consistency.

This recipe, covered tightly, will last for 2 days in the refrigerator.

YIELD: 4 baby servings, 2½ tablespoons (35 to 40 g) each

EACH SERVING CONTAINS: 31.9 calories; 1.1 g total fat; 0.5 grams saturated fat; 3.2 mg cholesterol; 5.4 mg sodium; 5.7 g carbohydrates; 0.7 g dietary fiber; 0.6 g protein; 24.4 mg calcium; 0.3 mg iron; 3769.5 IU vitamin A; and 8.5 mg vitamin C.

A Is for Acorn Squash Purée ❄

Acorn squash are easy to prepare. While they are frequently baked, they can also be roasted or microwaved. Their sweet-tasting flesh is rich in fiber.

1 acorn squash (about 1½ pounds [675 g])

2 to 4 tablespoons (28 to 60 ml) breast milk, formula, or apple juice

OVEN METHOD: Preheat the oven to 400°F (200°C, gas mark 6). Wash the squash, cut it in half, and remove the seeds and strings. Place each half cut side down in a shallow 8 x 11-inch (20 x 28 cm) baking dish with ¼ inch (6 mm) water. Bake 35 minutes, or until tender. Let cool. Scoop out the flesh from the skin. Purée in the blender with 2 to 4 tablespoons (28 to 60 ml) liquid from the pan (or breast milk, formula, or apple juice) for desired consistency.

This recipe, covered tightly, will last for 2 days in the refrigerator.

YIELD: 8 baby servings, 2 tablespoons (28 g) each

EACH SERVING (if using 4 tablespoons [60 ml] breast milk) CONTAINS: 39.4 calories; 0.4 g total fat; 0.2 grams saturated fat; 1.1 mg cholesterol; 3.9 mg sodium; 9.4 g carbohydrates; 1.3 g dietary fiber; 0.8 g protein; 30.5 mg calcium; 0.6 mg iron; 328.5 IU vitamin A; and 9.7 mg vitamin C.

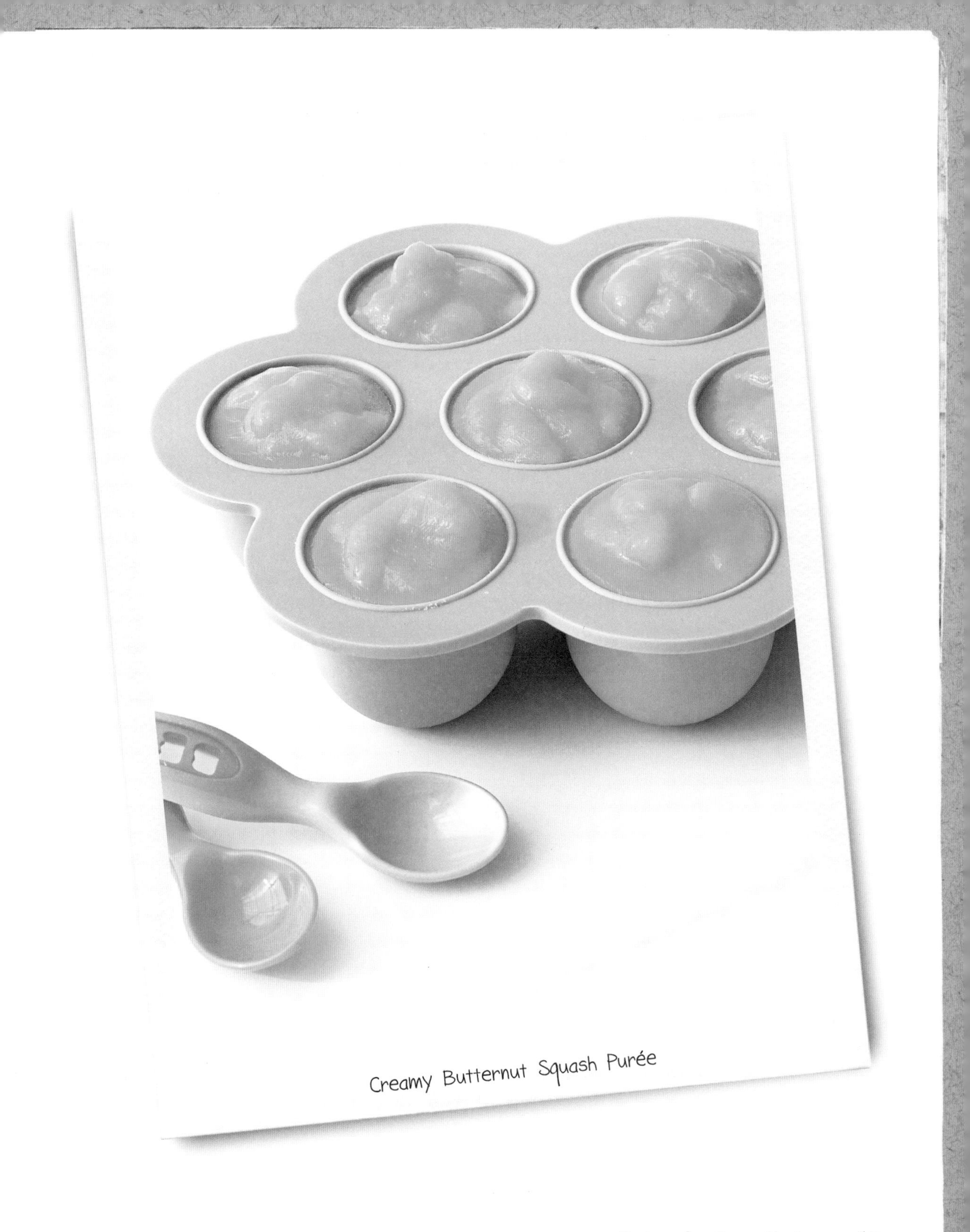

Creamy Butternut Squash Purée

Wee-licious Potato ❄

If your baby hesitates to eat this potato "pure," add a little sweet potato, apple, or pear purée. Sometimes, adding a favorite food to a new food makes babies more likely to accept what they are being given. (If you'd rather bake than microwave your potato, see next recipe.)

1 baking (russet or Idaho) potato

2 to 3 tablespoons (28 to 45 ml) breast milk or formula

MICROWAVE METHOD: Scrub the potato well. Prick the skin with a fork in several places. Microwave on high 10 minutes until soft. Let sit until cool enough to handle. Mash the potato flesh for your baby, adding breast milk or formula.

YIELD: 3 baby servings, 2 tablespoons (28 g) each

EACH SERVING (if using 3 tablespoons [45 ml] breast milk) CONTAINS: 81.1 calories; 0.8 g total fat; 0.3 grams saturated fat; 2.2 mg cholesterol; 10.2 mg sodium; 17.1 g carbohydrates; 1.7 g dietary fiber; 2.1 g protein; 16.3 mg calcium; 0.8 mg iron; 40.2 IU vitamin A; and 8.0 mg vitamin C.

Hot Potato!

Roasted potatoes or potatoes prepared in the microwave have twice as much vitamin C as peeled, boiled potatoes. That's because potatoes cooked with their skin on retain almost all of their nutrients.

Bun-in-the-Oven Baked Potato

When baking a potato in a conventional oven, don't wrap it in aluminum foil, as it creates moisture and steams the potato (the result will be similar to a boiled potato). But do bake several potatoes at once; you'll have enough for baby and the whole family!

1 baking (russet or Idaho) potato

Olive oil for coating (optional)

OVEN METHOD: Preheat the oven to 450°F (230°C, gas mark 8). Scrub the potato and pierce the skin two or three times with a fork. For a crispier skin, rub the potato with a light coating of olive oil. Place the potato directly on the middle oven rack. Bake 50 to 60 minutes or until soft or a fork easily pierces the potato.

YIELD: 3 baby servings, 2 tablespoons (28 g) each

EACH SERVING CONTAINS: 70.3 calories; 0.1 g total fat; 0.0 grams saturated fat; 0.0 mg cholesterol; 7.6 mg sodium; 16.0 g carbohydrates; 1.7 g dietary fiber; 1.9 g protein; 11.3 mg calcium; 0.8 mg iron; 7.6 IU vitamin A; and 7.3 mg vitamin C.

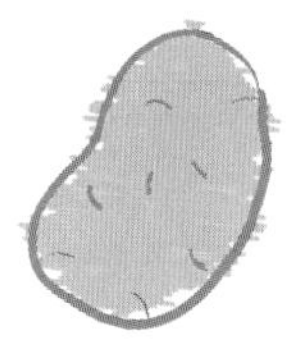

No-Cook Prune Purée

Prunes are sometimes called dried plums. In addition to being a source of iron and fiber, they contain an exceptional amount of the vitamins A and E. Homemade prune purée also has more than three times as much iron as the commercially prepared strained prunes with tapioca.

8 ready-to-serve dried, pitted plums

1/4 cup (60 ml) prune juice

1/4 cup (60 ml) pear nectar

Place all three ingredients in a blender. Purée until smooth.

This recipe, covered tightly, will last for 2 days in the refrigerator.

YIELD: 5 baby servings, 2 tablespoons (28 g) each

EACH SERVING CONTAINS: 44.0 calories; 0.0 g total fat; 0.0 grams saturated fat; 0.0 mg cholesterol; 5.3 mg sodium; 14.5 g carbohydrates; 1.0 g dietary fiber; 0.5 g protein; 1.6 mg calcium; 0.3 mg iron; 155.1 IU vitamin A; and 4.2 mg vitamin C.

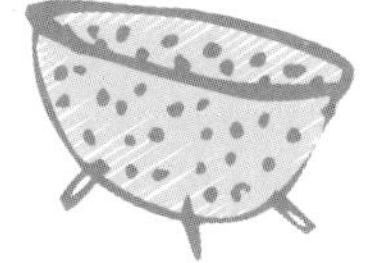

Power-Packed Prunes

Prunes can be found in the dried fruit section of most supermarkets. This recipe is delicious plain or mixed into oatmeal or other hot cereal.

12 ready-to-serve dried, pitted plums

1/4 cup (60 ml) water

1/4 cup (60 ml) prune juice

Peach or white grape juice (optional)

1/4 ripe mashed banana (optional)

Purée the plums in a blender until smooth. Add the water and prune juice (and peach or white grape juice and banana, if using). Purée until liquefied.

This recipe, covered tightly, will last for 3 days in the refrigerator.

YIELD: 4 baby servings, 4 tablespoons (55 g) each

EACH SERVING (if using no optional ingredients) CONTAINS: 115.6 calories; 0.0 g total fat; 0.0 grams saturated fat; 0.0 mg cholesterol; 2.2 mg sodium; 31.1 g carbohydrates; 3.2 g dietary fiber; 1.6 g protein; 1.3 mg calcium; 0.7 mg iron; 606.2 IU vitamin A; and 9.1 mg vitamin C.

Super P! No-Cook Purée

No-cook purées are made with raw fruit or vegetables, so no nutrients are lost through cooking. Prepare them just before serving for best consistency.

1 tablespoon (15 g) No-Cook Prune Purée (page 47)

1 tablespoon (15 g) Sweet Pear Purée (page 29)

Mix together purées and serve. For a creamier consistency, add 1 tablespoon (15 g) rice cereal to the fruit blend.

YIELD: 1 baby serving, or 2 tablespoons (28 g)

EACH SERVING CONTAINS: 39.2 calories; 0.1 g total fat; 0.0 grams saturated fat; 0.0 mg cholesterol; 3.0 mg sodium; 11.9 g carbohydrates; 1.4 g dietary fiber; 0.4 g protein; 3.5 mg calcium; 0.3 mg iron; 84.5 IU vitamin A; and 5.2 mg vitamin C.

Plums for Everyone!

For older children and adults, spread this purée on toast, bagels, pancakes, and waffles or use as a topping for yogurt, ice cream, rice pudding, or hot cereal.

Fuzzy Peach Purée

You can make this recipe with nectarines if you don't have peaches. Just peel them well and remove any white, stringy parts (near the core) before cooking.

1 small ripe peach

MICROWAVE METHOD: Halve and pit the peach. Place the peach halves cut side down on a microwave-safe plate and microwave on high 1 to 2 minutes until soft. Cool, remove the skin, and purée in a blender.

This recipe, covered tightly, will last for 2 days in the refrigerator.

YIELD: 1 baby serving, or 3 tablespoons (45 g)

EACH SERVING CONTAINS: 60.0 calories; 0.5 g total fat; 0.0 grams saturated fat; 0.0 mg cholesterol; 0.0 mg sodium; 15.0 g carbohydrates; 2.0 g dietary fiber; 1.0 g protein; 0.0 mg calcium; 0.4 mg iron; 300.0 IU vitamin A; and 9.0 mg vitamin C.

Plum Good Purée

Plums are a source of potassium for your baby. Potassium is a mineral that helps the kidneys function normally and maintains nerve and muscle activity throughout the body.

1 very ripe plum

¼ cup (60 ml) breast milk or formula

Peel, pit, and halve the plum and cut into small pieces. Place in blender with breast milk or formula. Purée until smooth, scraping down the sides of the blender as necessary.

YIELD: 4 baby servings, 2 tablespoons (28 g) each

EACH SERVING (if using breast milk) CONTAINS: 19.5 calories; 0.7 g total fat; 0.3 grams saturated fat; 2.2 mg cholesterol; 2.6 mg sodium; 3.4 g carbohydrates; 0.3 g dietary fiber; 0.3 g protein; 4.9 mg calcium; 0.1 mg iron; 82.7 IU vitamin A; and 1.5 mg vitamin C.

Peachy Plum

To sweeten this recipe even more, add some mashed banana or a little prune purée. Using the microwave to make this dish saves time.

1 sweet, ripe plum

1 small ripe peach

1 tablespoon to ½ cup (15 to 120 ml) water

MICROWAVE METHOD: Halve and pit the plum and peach. Place the halves cut side down on a microwave-safe plate and microwave on high 1 minute. Cool, remove skins, and purée in a blender. If the purée is too thick, thin with 1 or 2 tablespoons (15 to 28 ml) water.

STOVETOP METHOD: Blanch the peach and plum in boiling water 10 to 15 seconds. With a slotted spoon, remove from the water, cool, peel, quarter, and pit the fruit. Combine the fruit and ½ cup (120 ml) water in a saucepan over medium-high heat and bring to a boil. Reduce the heat and simmer 5 to 10 minutes (depending on the ripeness of the fruit) until soft. Allow mixture to cool and purée the fruit with ¼ cup (60 ml) of the cooking liquid in a blender for 30 seconds. Add more liquid as needed.

YIELD: 4 baby servings, 2 tablespoons (28 g) each

EACH SERVING CONTAINS: 23.8 calories; 0.1 g total fat; 0.0 grams saturated fat; 0.0 mg cholesterol; 0.0 mg sodium; 6.1 g carbohydrates; 0.8 g dietary fiber; 0.4 g protein; 0.0 mg calcium; 0.1 mg iron; 125.0 IU vitamin A; and 3.0 mg vitamin C.

Fuss-Free Pumpkin and Banana Purée ❄

Pumpkin is a very healthy source of beta carotene, vitamin C, and folate. While you're welcome to prepare the pumpkin on your own, it's much easier (and equally healthy) to use pure canned pumpkin. Look for it in the baking aisle; just be sure not to grab the "pumpkin pie" mix by mistake, because that contains sugar and other additives you don't want to give your baby.

1/4 cup (60 g) 100 percent pure pumpkin

1/2 small banana

Mash pumpkin with banana.

This recipe, covered tightly, will last for 2 days in the refrigerator.

YIELD: 3 baby servings, 2 tablespoons (28 g) each

EACH SERVING CONTAINS: 24.2 calories; 0.2 g total fat; 0.0 grams saturated fat; 0.0 mg cholesterol; 1.0 mg sodium; 6.0 g carbohydrates; 1.3 g dietary fiber; 0.6 g protein; 4.3 mg calcium; 0.2 mg iron; 2929.3 IU vitamin A; and 1.7 mg vitamin C.

Yummy Recipe Tip: Pumpkin Makes a Perfect Pair!

There are so many foods that complement the flavor of pumpkin. Feel free to experiment by mixing any one of these foods with pumpkin purée for a totally new meal:

- Acorn Squash
- Apples
- Bananas
- Butternut Squash
- Chicken
- Peaches
- Yogurt

Peach and Banana Whip

Peaches can have either a white or yellow flesh; those with white flesh tend to be sweeter and less acidic. Either variety will work, though, as long as they're ripe.

1 small ripe peach

2 tablespoons (28 g) mashed, ripe banana

1 tablespoon (15 ml) breast milk or formula

MICROWAVE METHOD: Halve and pit the peach. Place it cut sides down on a microwave-safe plate and microwave on high 1 minute. When cool enough to handle, remove the skin. Purée the peach and banana in a blender. Remove and whisk in the breast milk or formula with a fork.

YIELD: 3 baby servings, 2 heaping tablespoons (30 to 40 g) each

EACH SERVING CONTAINS: 31.9 calories; 0.4 g total fat; 0.1 grams saturated fat; 0.7 mg cholesterol; 1.0 mg sodium; 7.5 g carbohydrates; 0.9 g dietary fiber; 0.5 g protein; 2.1 mg calcium; 0.2 mg iron; 116.9 IU vitamin A; and 4.1 mg vitamin C.

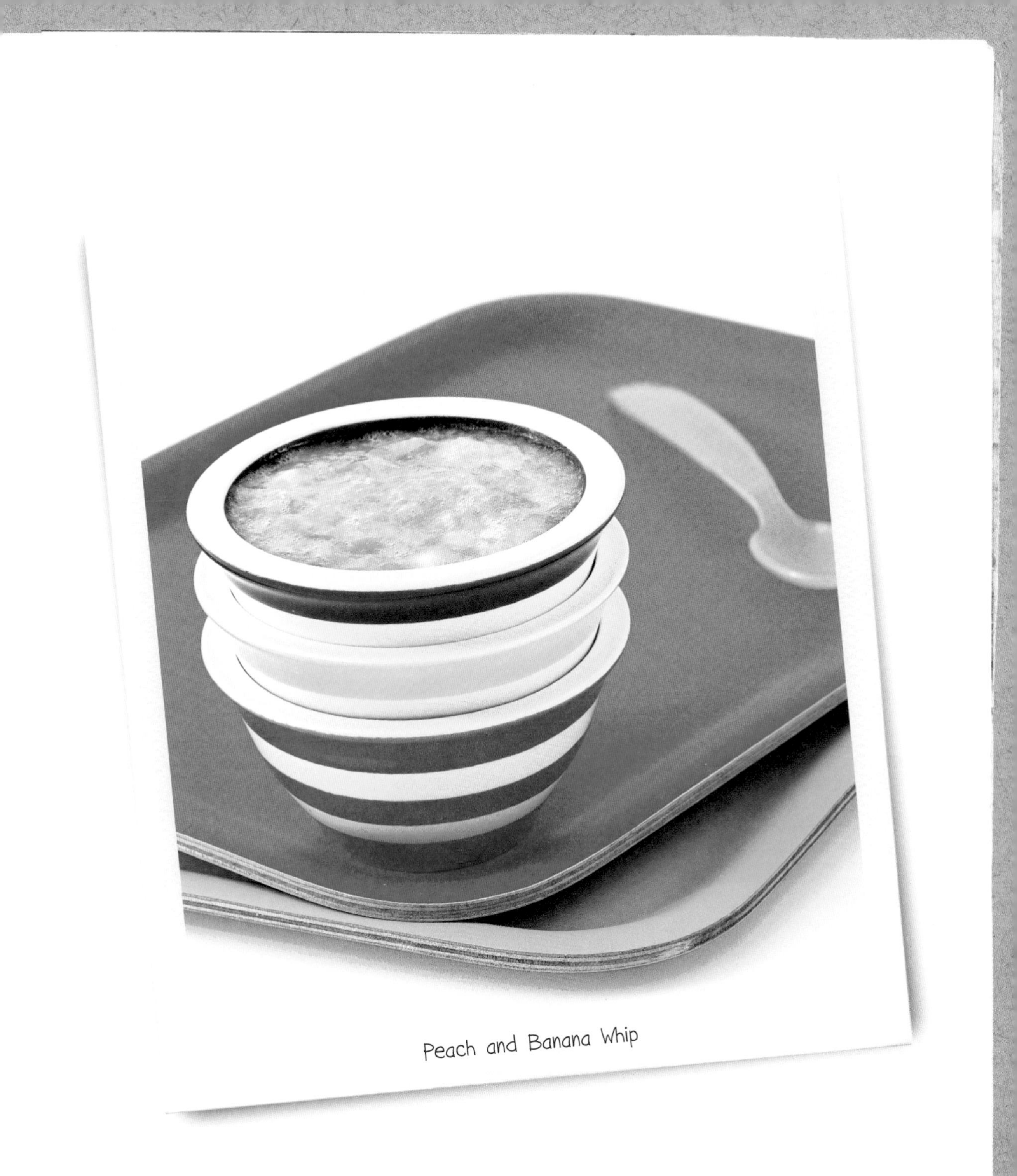

Peach and Banana Whip

Prune-Apple-Banana Smoothie

This trio of fruit is unbeatable for flavor and nutrition—it packs vitamin C, potassium, fiber, and fantastic taste! Everyone in the family will want one.

¼ cup (60 g) unsweetened applesauce

¼ cup (60 ml) prune juice

⅓ small banana

Combine all ingredients in blender and process until smooth.

YIELD: 4 baby servings, 2 tablespoons (28 g) each

EACH SERVING CONTAINS: 26.5 calories; 0.1 g total fat; 0.0 grams saturated fat; 0.0 mg cholesterol; 1.0 mg sodium; 6.8 g carbohydrates; 0.6 g dietary fiber; 0.2 g protein; 3.0 mg calcium; 0.3 mg iron; 11.2 IU vitamin A; and 1.8 mg vitamin C.

Peachy-Keen Banana Purée

The beautiful, bright color of this recipe will be very appealing to baby. To save time, you can also use jarred or canned peaches packed in their natural juices, not heavy syrup.

½ cup peaches

⅓ banana

Peel, pit, and cook peaches. Combine with banana in blender and process until smooth.

YIELD: 2 baby servings, 2 tablespoons (28 g) each

EACH SERVING CONTAINS: 32.1 calories; 0.2 g total fat; 0.0 grams saturated fat; 0.0 mg cholesterol; 0.2 mg sodium; 8.1 g carbohydrates; 1.1 g dietary fiber; 0.6 g protein; 3.2 mg calcium; 0.1 mg iron; 134.8 IU vitamin A; and 4.2 mg vitamin C.

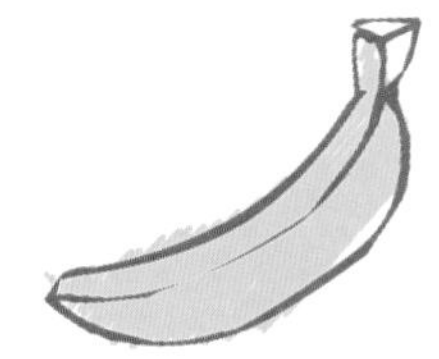

A to B Apple-Butternut Squash Purée ❄

Mixing together fruit and vegetable purées is a good way to help babies develop a taste for vegetables. If you don't have apple purée on hand, try pear, apricot, or peach purée. And if you'd like to make a larger batch to freeze, just remember the 1:1 ratio.

1 tablespoon (15 g) Perfect Apple Purée (page 29)

1 tablespoon (15 g) Creamy Butternut Squash Purée (page 44)

Mix together purées and serve.

YIELD: 1 baby serving, or 2 tablespoons (28 g)

EACH SERVING CONTAINS: 20.3 calories; 0.6 g total fat; 0.3 grams saturated fat; 1.6 mg cholesterol; 2.7 mg sodium; 4.1 g carbohydrates; 0.6 g dietary fiber; 0.4 g protein; 12.7 mg calcium; 0.2 mg iron; 1889.3 IU vitamin A; and 4.7 mg vitamin C.

Green Pea and Potato Garden Purée ❄

The texture of starchy vegetables makes them excellent first foods for baby because they purée into a very smooth paste that is easy for your little one to "chew" with his lips and gums.

1 tablespoon (15 g) More Green Peas Purée, Please! (page 39)

1 tablespoon (15 g) Wee-licious Potato (page 46)

Mash together ingredients and serve. For a creamier consistency, add a bit of breast milk or formula.

YIELD: 1 baby serving, or 2 tablespoons (28 g)

EACH SERVING CONTAINS: 77.0 calories; 0.6 g total fat; 0.2 grams saturated fat; 1.5 mg cholesterol; 5.6 mg sodium; 11.7 g carbohydrates; 1.9 g dietary fiber; 2.1 g protein; 9.3 mg calcium; 0.7 mg iron; 125.1 IU vitamin A; and 5.7 mg vitamin C.

Make Fresh-Cooked Squash in Minutes!

The following are some other options for cooking squash. If you have leftovers, add the flesh or purée to the family meal; it tastes especially delicious in soups and pastas.

- *Butternut squash:* Cut the squash in half and remove seeds and membranes. Place cut sides down in a microwave-safe dish. Add 1/2 cup (120 ml) water and microwave on high 12 to 15 minutes until tender. Cool and remove the flesh.
- *Acorn squash:* Microwave the whole squash on high 1 minute. Allow to cool; then cut in half and remove seeds and membranes. Place cut sides down in a microwave-safe dish. Add 1/4 cup (60 ml) water and microwave on high 8 to 10 minutes or until tender. Cool and remove the flesh.

TOTALLY TUBULAR NEW TEXTURES:

RECIPES FOR EIGHT MONTHS

Eight months is an age of self-discovery and exploration. Your baby may want to play with his food, feel it, squish it, smell it, taste it, spit it out—and occasionally eat it.

Of course, you'll still be doing most of the spoon-feeding at this stage, but encourage your little one's independence and try to sense how much you should help. This is a good age for your baby to join you at the dining table in a high chair.

Finally, while finger food and self-feeding will have lots of appeal, your baby should still be getting three to four feedings of breast milk or formula (24 to 32 ounces [700 to 950 ml] total) each day. Since this remains your baby's primary source of nutrition, continue with these feedings as part of your normal routine.

Helpful Hints for the High Chair

The following are some reminders and recommendations for preparing food for your eight-month-old:

- Serve ¼ cup (55 g) single-grain baby cereal twice a day.
- Offer 2 tablespoons (28 g) of vegetables rich in vitamins A and C twice a day. (Vegetables should be washed, peeled/seeded, and cooked.)
- Offer 2 tablespoons (28 g) of fruit rich in vitamins A and C twice a day. The texture can now be thicker and chunkier. (Wash, peel, core, and seed very ripe fruit. Mash or cut into thin, small pieces and serve as finger food.)
- Serve ½ cup (120 ml) diluted juice rich in vitamins A and C once daily. All liquids at mealtime should be offered in a two-handled sippy cup. The ones without valves work best, but you may want to try others.
- Do not add salt, sugar, honey, or seasoning to your baby's foods.
- Do not force-feed your baby.
- Never leave your child unattended when eating or drinking.
- Continue to introduce one new food at a time, every three days.

NEW BITES FOR YOUR EIGHT-MONTH-OLD

At eight months, your baby may have a few teeth starting to appear. Since up-and-down chewing movements are developing, you can start to offer your baby soft, chunky food to encourage the development of this skill. It is fine to continue serving mashed and puréed food, as well.

You can make these additions to your baby's diet, in addition to incorporating what she already enjoys from the previous sections:

VEGETABLES (cooked)	• Carrots • String beans • Wax beans
FRUITS	• Very ripe, fresh apricots • Dried, unsulphured apricots* • Blueberries
JUICE	• Apricot • Carrot
FINGER FOOD/OTHER	• Baby crackers (oat or rice) • Cooked rice noodles, cut into small pieces • Cooked rice or barley • Full-fat cottage cheese** • Hard-cooked egg yolk*** • Pieces of peeled soft fruit (fresh or cooked) • Plain oat Cheerios • Ripe banana slices • Soft cooked vegetable pieces

* Unsulphured apricots are dark brown in color and have a sweet, caramel flavor. They do not contain sulphur dioxide, a preservative that gives dried apricots their bright orange color.

** Be sure to serve baby whole-milk cottage cheese, not the reduced-fat or fat-free variety.

*** Pediatricians suggest you wait to serve cooked egg whites to your baby until after his first birthday. Allergic reactions to egg whites are very common, so it's best to wait until your child has grown older before introducing them. Leftover cooked egg whites can be used in tuna or egg salad or other cooked dishes for family and toddlers a year and older.

Naturally Sweet Apricot Purée

Be sure to buy unsulphured dried apricots, which are brownish-orange in color. Their bright-orange counterparts, which are treated with sulfur-containing preservatives, may be sensitive to baby.

½ cup (65 g) dried apricots

1 cup (235 ml) water

MICROWAVE METHOD: Combine the apricots and water in a microwave-safe dish, cover with a lid, and microwave on high 5 minutes. Allow to cool and then transfer mixture to a blender. Purée for 2 minutes.

STOVETOP METHOD: Bring the dried apricots and water to a boil in a small saucepan over medium heat. Cover, reduce heat, and simmer 30 minutes, or until the apricots are soft.

Allow mixture to cool and then purée with cooking water in a blender until smooth.

This recipe, covered tightly, will last for 2 days in the refrigerator.

YIELD: 4 baby servings, 2 tablespoons (28 g) each

EACH SERVING CONTAINS: 42.6 calories; 0.0 g total fat; 0.0 grams saturated fat; 0.0 mg cholesterol; 1.9 mg sodium; 9.7 g carbohydrates; 0.8 g dietary fiber; 0.4 g protein; 7.7 mg calcium; 0.7 mg iron; 967.3 IU vitamin A; and 0.0 mg vitamin C.

Four-Fruit Compote

Pitted prunes, commonly packaged as "dried plums," can be found in the dried fruit aisle of your grocery store.

¼ cup (44 g) prunes (dried plums)

¼ cup (33 g) dried apricots

1 apple

1 pear

2 cups (475 ml) water

STOVETOP METHOD: Dice the prunes and apricots. Peel, core, and dice the apple and pear. Place the prunes, apricots, apple, pear, and water in a small saucepan. Bring to a boil, reduce heat, and simmer 20 to 30 minutes until the fruit is soft and most of the water is absorbed. Stir occasionally to prevent sticking and add more water if needed. Mash and serve warm.

YIELD: 2 baby servings, ⅓ cup (85 g) each

EACH SERVING CONTAINS: 161.6 calories; 0.2 g total fat; 0.0 grams saturated fat; 0.0 mg cholesterol; 7.9 mg sodium; 40.8 g carbohydrates; 5.8 g dietary fiber; 1.0 g protein; 25.9 mg calcium; 1.1 mg iron; 1127.7 IU vitamin A; and 7.8 mg vitamin C.

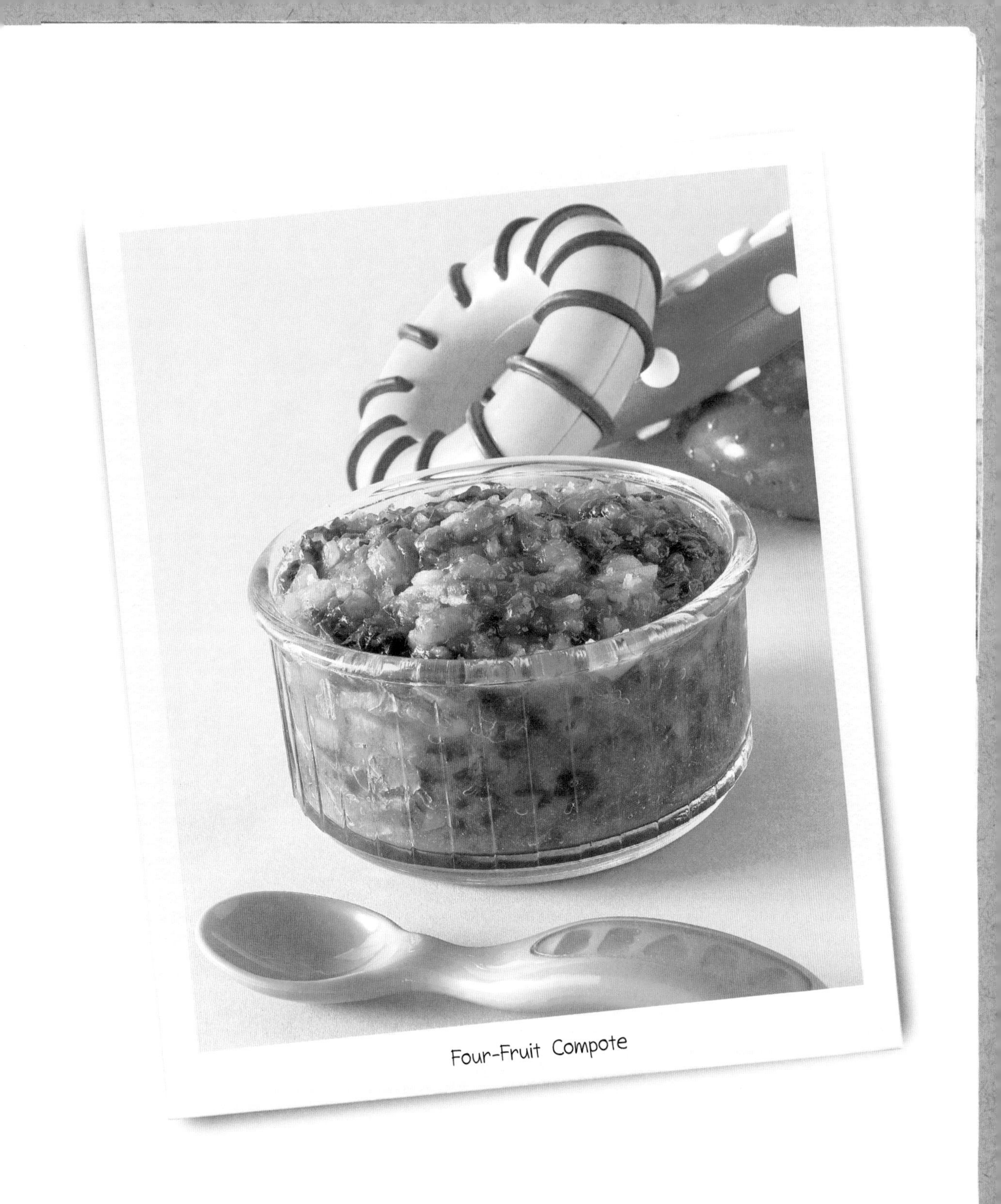

Four-Fruit Compote

Bright Eyes Mashed Carrots

Ready-to-eat baby carrots are available in grocery stores and markets. Be sure they don't have any preservatives and always rinse them—even if they're packaged as "ready-to-eat."

4 baby carrots

1 tablespoon to 1⁄4 cup (15 to 60 ml) water

MICROWAVE METHOD: Wash and dice carrots and place them in a small glass bowl with 1 tablespoon (15 ml) water. Cover and microwave on high 2 minutes. Allow to cool slightly and then purée in a blender or mash with a fork. Add apple juice, breast milk, or formula if needed to achieve desired consistency.

STOVETOP METHOD: Place carrots in a saucepan with 1⁄4 cup (60 ml) water. Bring to a boil, cover, reduce the heat, and simmer 10 minutes or until carrots are soft. Allow to cool slightly and then purée in a blender or mash with a fork. Add apple juice, breast milk, or formula if needed to achieve desired consistency.

YIELD: 1 to 2 baby servings, 2 tablespoons (28 g) each

EACH SERVING CONTAINS: 6.7 calories; 0.0 g total fat; 0.0 grams saturated fat; 0.0 mg cholesterol; 7.5 mg sodium; 1.5 g carbohydrates; 0.3 g dietary fiber; 0.2 g protein; 3.3 mg calcium; 0.0 mg iron; 2083.3 IU vitamin A; and 1.0 mg vitamin C.

Puréed Carrots with Pretty Pears

The texture of whipped carrots is a favorite among babies. Combined with pears and they'll enjoy this healthy meal even more.

4 baby carrots

1⁄4 pear

3 tablespoons (45 ml) water

MICROWAVE METHOD: Cut the carrots lengthwise, then in half, and place in a small glass bowl. Peel, core, and chop the pear and add to bowl. Add water. Cover and microwave on high 2 minutes. Allow to cool slightly and then purée in a blender. Add apple juice, breast milk, or formula if needed to achieve desired consistency.

YIELD: 2 to 4 baby servings, 2 tablespoons (28 g) each

EACH SERVING CONTAINS: 16.2 calories; 0.0 g total fat; 0.0 grams saturated fat; 0.0 mg cholesterol; 4.0 mg sodium; 4.2 g carbohydrates; 0.9 g dietary fiber; 0.2 g protein; 3.7 mg calcium; 0.0 mg iron; 1046.8 IU vitamin A; and 1.4 mg vitamin C.

Any Way You Please Potato and Peas ❄

Peas may be tiny, but they're big on nutrition, contributing calcium, iron, and vitamins A and C to the diet. Frozen peas are just as nutritious as fresh, so don't hesitate to use them when making baby food.

1/4 cup (35 g) green peas, thawed and drained

2 tablespoons (28 g) flesh from Bun-in-the-Oven Baked Potato (page 46)

MICROWAVE METHOD: Cook the peas in a microwave-safe dish according to package directions. Place in blender with cooking liquid and baked potato flesh and purée. If a thinner purée is desired, add breast milk or formula as needed.

YIELD: 2 baby servings, 2 tablespoons (28 g) each

EACH SERVING CONTAINS: 28.4 calories; 0.1 g total fat; 0.0 grams saturated fat; 0.0 mg cholesterol; 19.3 mg sodium; 5.9 g carbohydrates; 1.1 g dietary fiber; 1.2 g protein; 4.7 mg calcium; 0.4 mg iron; 344.7 IU vitamin A; and 4.8 mg vitamin C.

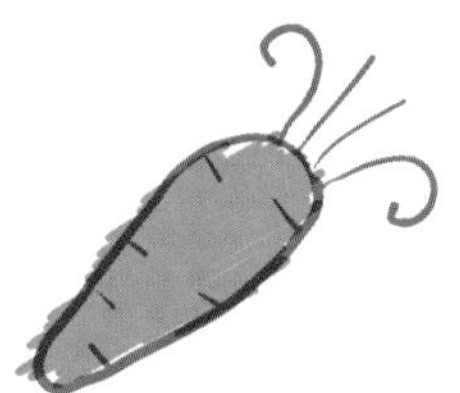

Orange You Cute Carrots and Sweet Potato ❄

This combination is loaded with beta carotene, a powerful antioxidant that gives carrots and sweet potatoes their bright orange color.

4 baby carrots

1/4 cup (56 g) peeled, cubed, and cooked sweet potato

3 tablespoons (45 ml) water

MICROWAVE METHOD: Cut the carrots lengthwise, then in half, and place in a small glass bowl with the cooked sweet potato and water. Cover and microwave on high 2 minutes. Allow to cool slightly and then purée in a blender or mash with a fork. Use apple juice, breast milk, or formula if needed to achieve desired consistency.

YIELD: 4 baby servings, 2 tablespoons (28 g) each

EACH SERVING CONTAINS: 12.8 calories; 0.0 g total fat; 0.0 grams saturated fat; 0.0 mg cholesterol; 7.1 mg sodium; 3.0 g carbohydrates; 0.5 g dietary fiber; 0.3 g protein; 5.0 mg calcium; 0.1 mg iron; 3009.2 IU vitamin A; and 2.1 mg vitamin C.

Yummy Recipe Tip: Carrots Make Great Finger Food

Baby carrots can also be cut in thin strips (julienned) and microwaved, steamed, or simmered until very soft and served as finger food. When cooked or served with a little unsalted butter, the fat helps the body absorb the carrots' vitamin A.

My First Cheese, Please!

Cheeses are typically first offered to the non-allergic baby between eight and ten months of age. For those infants who do not have a lot of experience with textures and lumpy foods, whirl the cottage cheese in the blender first.

½ small avocado

⅓ small banana

¼ cup (55 g) whole milk cottage cheese

½ cup (120 ml) breast milk or formula

Scoop out the flesh from the avocado and place in blender with banana, cottage cheese, and breast milk or formula. Purée well.

YIELD: 6 baby servings, 2 tablespoons (28 g) each

EACH SERVING (if using breast milk) CONTAINS: 57.0 calories; 3.8 g total fat; 1.0 grams saturated fat; 5.0 mg cholesterol; 41.4 mg sodium; 4.8 g carbohydrates; 1.3 g dietary fiber; 1.6 g protein; 15.9 mg calcium; 0.1 mg iron; 88.9 IU vitamin A; and 3.3 mg vitamin C.

Better-for-Baby Sweet Potato "Fries"

These beat regular French fries in both taste and nutrition since they contain more vitamins and minerals than traditional fries. They also make a good snack or finger food for the whole family!

1 large sweet potato

1 to 2 tablespoons (15 to 28 ml) olive oil

OVEN METHOD: Preheat the oven to 400°F (200°C, gas mark 6). Peel the sweet potato, cut it in half, then into ¼-inch (6-mm) thick slices, and again into ¼-inch (6-mm) sticks. Put in a large bowl, add the oil, and toss until coated with oil. Place on a baking sheet. (Alternatively, arrange sweet potato sticks in a single layer on a baking sheet and spray with olive oil.) Bake on the middle rack 10 minutes. Turn the potatoes and bake 10 minutes more.

YIELD: 8 to 10 fries, or 4 to 5 servings, 2 fries each

EACH SERVING (if using 2 tablespoons [28 ml] of olive oil) CONTAINS: 35.8 calories; 5.6 g total fat; 0.8 grams saturated fat; 0.0 mg cholesterol; 8.2 mg sodium; 5.4 g carbohydrates; 0.8 g dietary fiber; 0.4 g protein; 8.2 mg calcium; 0.2 mg iron; 4753.5 IU vitamin A; and 3.9 mg vitamin C.

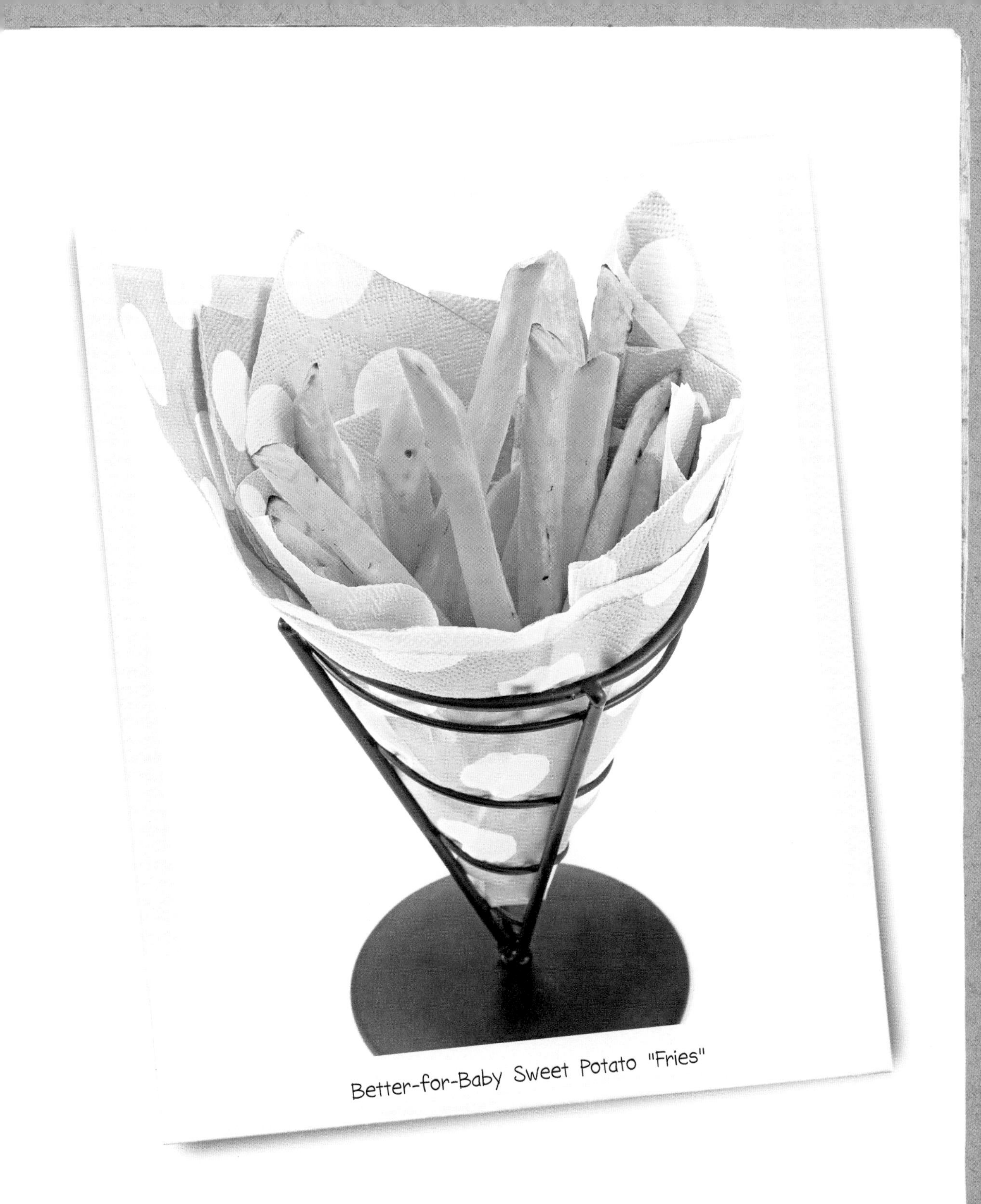

Better-for-Baby Sweet Potato "Fries"

Buttered with Love Green Beans

Green beans are a good source of vitamins and minerals, including iron and vitamins A, C, and K. If you don't have green beans on hand, you can use yellow wax beans or purple beans in this recipe.

6 green beans (about 1/4 cup [25 g])

1/2 cup (120 ml) water

1 teaspoon unsalted butter

STOVETOP METHOD: Wash and trim beans and then cut into thin strips. Bring water to boil in a small saucepan and add the beans. Cook 5 minutes. Allow to cool slightly and then place the beans, water, and butter into a blender and purée.

YIELD: 1 baby serving, or 2 1/2 tablespoons (35 to 40 g)

EACH SERVING CONTAINS: 40.7 calories; 3.7 g total fat; 2.7 grams saturated fat; 10.0 mg cholesterol; 2.9 mg sodium; 1.9 g carbohydrates; 0.6 g dietary fiber; 0.3 g protein; 5.9 mg calcium; 0.1 mg iron; 192.1 IU vitamin A; and 0.4 mg vitamin C.

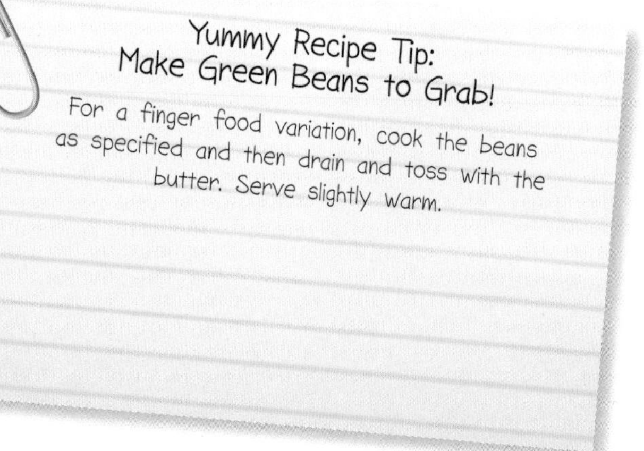

Mighty Tasty Blueberry and Pear Mash

Blueberries are among the fruit with the highest antioxidant activity and are often called a "superfood" due to their significant health benefits.

1/2 large pear

2 tablespoons (18 g) blueberries

2 tablespoons (28 ml) water

STOVETOP METHOD: Peel, core, seed, and chop pear. Place in saucepan with blueberries and water and simmer for 7 minutes or until fruit begins to break down. Allow mixture to cool slightly and then transfer to blender and whip until smooth. Strain (to remove skins from the blueberries), cool, and serve.

YIELD: 4 baby servings, 2 tablespoons (28 g) each

EACH SERVING CONTAINS: 15.5 calories; 0.0 g total fat; 0.0 grams saturated fat; 0.0 mg cholesterol; 0.3 mg sodium; 4.1 g carbohydrates; 0.8 g dietary fiber; 0.1 g protein; 2.3 mg calcium; 0.1 mg iron; 7.6 IU vitamin A; and 1.4 mg vitamin C.

Basmati Baby Rice

This recipe will help broaden your baby's palate by introducing him to a new flavor—a nutty aromatic one that he just might love!

½ cup (80 g) cooked basmati rice

¼ cup (60 ml) breast milk or formula

Place the cooked rice in a blender with the breast milk or formula and blend 45 seconds.

YIELD: 5 baby servings, 2 tablespoons (28 g) each

EACH SERVING (if using breast milk) CONTAINS: 23.6 calories; 0.6 g total fat; 0.3 grams saturated fat; 1.7 mg cholesterol; 48.1 mg sodium; 4.3 g carbohydrates; 0.1 g dietary fiber; 0.4 g protein; 3.9 mg calcium; 0.0 mg iron; 126.1 IU vitamin A; and 0.7 mg vitamin C.

Comfy and Cozy Rice and Apricot Pudding

This recipe is extremely versatile. For variety, try replacing the apricot with No Cook Prune Purée (page 47), mashed banana, Perfect Apple Purée (page 29), Sweet Pear Purée (page 29), Fuzzy Peach Purée (48), Plum Good Purée (page 49), or Oh So Sweet Potato Purée (page 34).

½ cup (80 g) cooked basmati rice

¼ cup (55 g) Naturally Sweet Apricot Purée (page 56)

¼ cup (60 ml) breast milk or formula

Mix the rice and apricot purée with the breast milk or formula. If a creamier consistency is desired, add more liquid.

YIELD: 5 baby servings, 2 tablespoons (28 g) each

EACH SERVING CONTAINS: 28.1 calories; 0.6 g total fat; 0.2 grams saturated fat; 1.6 mg cholesterol; 46.0 mg sodium; 5.3 g carbohydrates; 0.2 g dietary fiber; 0.5 g protein; 4.8 mg calcium; 4.8 mg iron; 248.2 IU vitamin A; and 0.7 mg vitamin C.

Eggs for All Occasions

Eggs provide protein, vitamin A, B vitamins, calcium, phosphorus, iron, and zinc. By their eighth month, babies may be given well-cooked, mashed, hard-cooked egg yolks mixed with other age-appropriate foods (such as the rice above). One-year-olds may be given whole eggs, provided that there is no history of egg allergies in the family.

Positively Perfect Pumpkin and Pears ❄

In a pinch, you can just serve baby the pumpkin purée on its own for a healthy, nutrient-rich meal. For more delicious recipe ideas using pumpkin purée, see page 50.

1 ripe pear

1/4 cup (61 g) pumpkin purée (fresh or canned)

1/4 cup (60 ml) pear nectar or unsweetened apple juice

Peel, core, and dice pear. Put all ingredients into a blender and purée until smooth.

YIELD: 4 servings, 2 tablespoons (28 g) each

EACH SERVING (if using pear nectar) CONTAINS: 39.9 calories; 0.1 g total fat; 0.0 grams saturated fat; 0.0 mg cholesterol; 1.5 mg sodium; 10.2 g carbohydrates; 2.0 g dietary fiber; 0.4 g protein; 10.0 mg calcium; 0.2 mg iron; 2197.7 IU vitamin A; and 4.5 mg vitamin C.

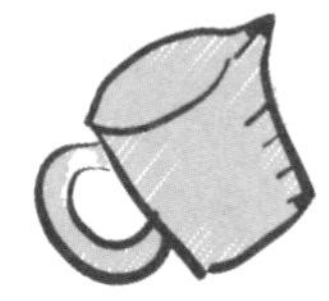

Healthy Baby Tip: Juicy Insight You Should Know

Large amounts of fruit or juice may make an infant's stool acidic and irritating to the skin. This can result in a painful red rash, which may be mistaken for an allergic reaction. Since most fruit juice also contains a lot of sugar, your baby may get diarrhea from drinking too much of it. Again, juice is best in small amounts. Since juice is a rich source of vitamin C, it can help with iron uptake when consumed alongside a meal; however, it should be served to baby diluted and limited to 4 ounces (1/2 cup [120 ml]) daily.

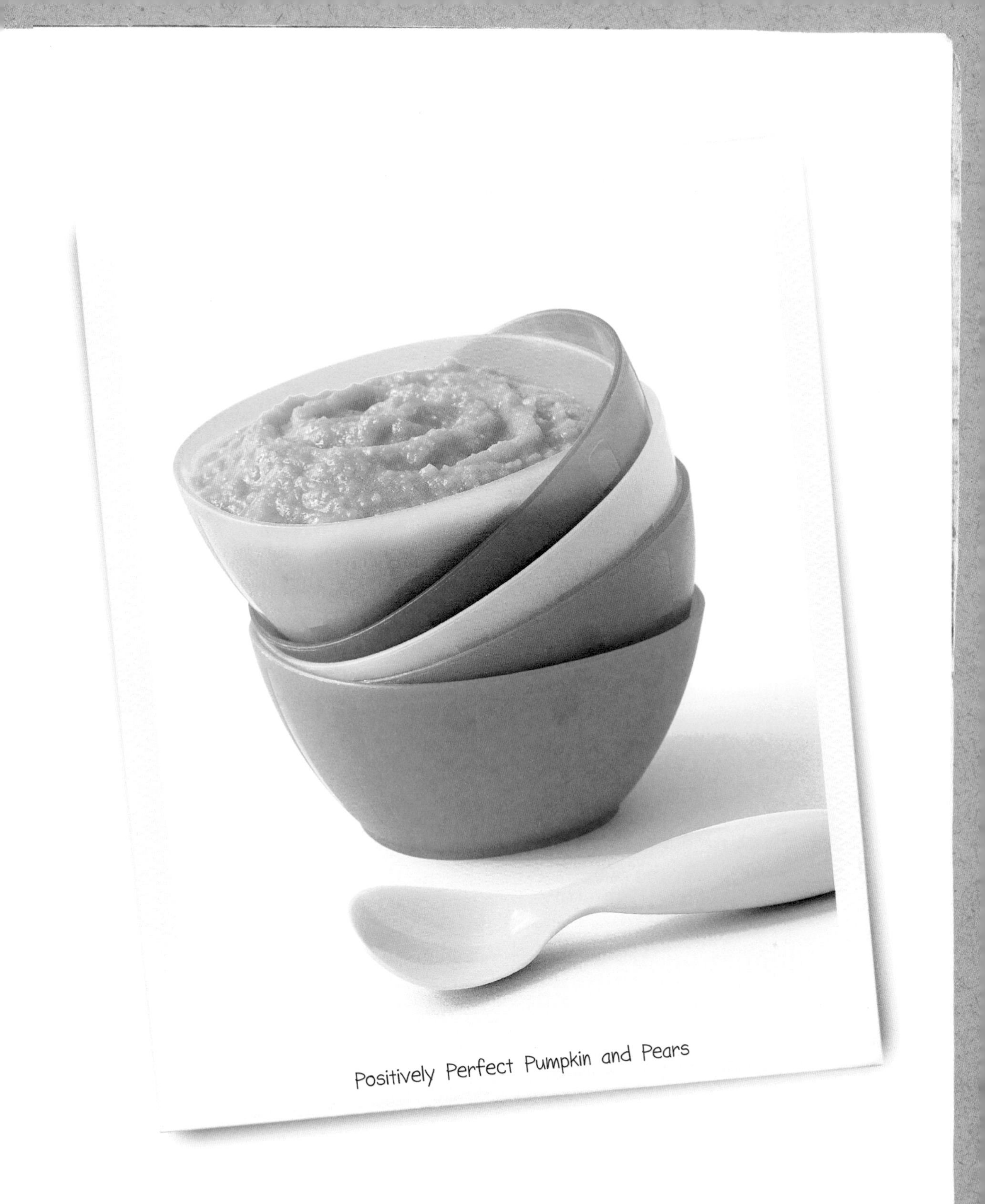

Positively Perfect Pumpkin and Pears

Color Me Orange Carrot-Potato Purée ❄

Root vegetables always purée nicely in a blender and freeze exceptionally well. This recipe should be among your frozen staples and was designed to produce a larger yield for that purpose.

3 small potatoes

1 cup (130 g) chopped carrots

1 cup (235 ml) water

1 tablespoon (14 g) butter

STOVETOP METHOD: Peel and cube the potatoes. Place with the carrots in a small saucepan with the water. Cover and bring to a boil. Reduce heat and simmer 25 minutes until the vegetables are soft. Drain. Whisk in the butter. Take out baby's portion, and freeze the rest for later.

YIELD: 12 servings, 2 tablespoons (28 g) each

EACH SERVING CONTAINS: 46.1 calories; 1.0 g total fat; 0.7 grams saturated fat; 2.5 mg cholesterol; 12.2 mg sodium; 8.4 g carbohydrates; 1.1 g dietary fiber; 1.0 g protein; 9.7 mg calcium; 0.4 mg iron; 1818.8 IU vitamin A; and 5.1 mg vitamin C.

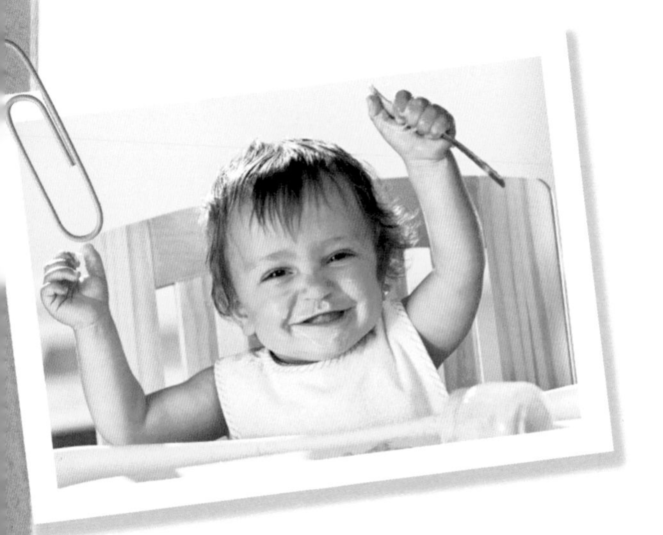

Creamy Cottage Cheese and Carrot Purée

The creamy texture and savory taste of cottage cheese goes well with puréed carrots.

4 baby carrots

1 tablespoon (15 ml) water

1/4 cup (55 g) whole milk cottage cheese

MICROWAVE METHOD: Cut the carrots lengthwise, then in half, and place in a small microwave-safe bowl with water. Cover and microwave on high for 2 minutes. Cool slightly and then purée in a blender or mash with a fork. Add cottage cheese and blend well.

YIELD: 2 baby servings, 2 tablespoons (28 g) each

EACH SERVING CONTAINS: 35.8 calories; 1.3 g total fat; 0.8 grams saturated fat; 6.3 mg cholesterol; 117.5 mg sodium; 2.5 g carbohydrates; 0.3 g dietary fiber; 3.2 g protein; 23.3 mg calcium; 0.0 mg iron; 883.3 IU vitamin A; and 0.2 mg vitamin C.

Bananas in the Snow

Being a very rich source of calcium and protein makes cottage cheese a good food for baby. This recipe also tastes great spread on wheat toast for adults!

1/4 small ripe banana

1/4 cup (55 g) whole milk cottage cheese

Mash banana with a fork and combine with cottage cheese.

YIELD: 3 baby servings, 2 tablespoons (28 g) each

EACH SERVING CONTAINS: 37.5 calories; 0.9 g total fat; 0.5 grams saturated fat; 4.2 mg cholesterol; 73.5 mg sodium; 5.5 g carbohydrates; 0.5 g dietary fiber; 2.2 g protein; 14.3 mg calcium; 0.1 mg iron; 45.9 IU vitamin A; and 1.7 mg vitamin C.

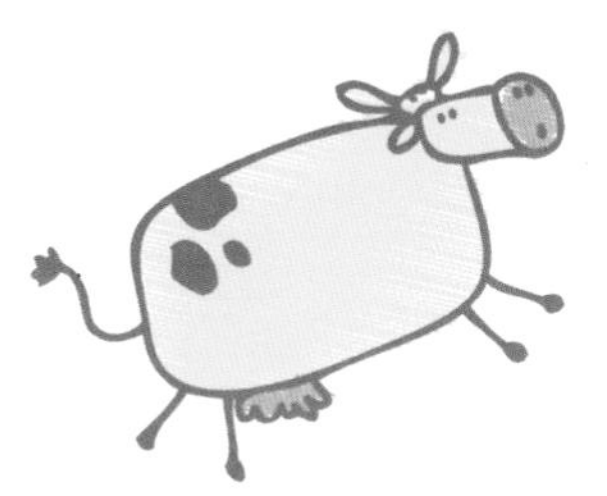

Blueberry and Banana Breakfast

The nutritional value of blueberries makes them one of the best foods we can eat. When your baby can handle finger foods, try cutting blueberries in half for a healthy snack.

1/4 cup (36 g) blueberries

2 tablespoons (28 ml) water

1/3 large banana

STOVETOP METHOD: Put the blueberries into a saucepan with water and cook for 3 minutes or until the fruit starts to break open. Mash fruit with the back of a spoon. Cool slightly and pour mixture into blender. Add banana and purée until smooth. Press through sieve if necessary to remove blueberry skins. Cool and serve.

YIELD: 3 baby servings, 2 tablespoons (28 g) each

EACH SERVING CONTAINS: 18.7 calories; 0.0 g total fat; 0.0 grams saturated fat; 0.0 mg cholesterol; 0.3 mg sodium; 4.8 g carbohydrates; 0.6 g dietary fiber; 0.2 g protein; 1.4 mg calcium; 0.1 mg iron; 15.1 IU vitamin A; and 2.3 mg vitamin C.

Summertime Watermelon Mash

Sweet, juicy watermelon is a concentrated source of vitamin C. It's also about 90 percent water, so it's easy for baby to digest.

5 cubes (1-inch or 2.5 cm) of seedless watermelon

½ small banana

Whirl ingredients in a blender until smooth.

YIELD: 4 baby servings, 2 tablespoons (28 g) each

EACH SERVING CONTAINS: 18.1 calories; 0.5 g total fat; 0.0 grams saturated fat; 0.0 mg cholesterol; 0.7 mg sodium; 5.1 carbohydrates; 0.5 g dietary fiber; 0.2 g protein; 2.0 mg calcium; 0.1 mg iron; 72.0 IU vitamin A; and 2.2 mg vitamin C.

That's Beta-Carotene on My Bib! Carrots with Apricots

Both carrots and apricots are very healthy and full of beta-carotene, which gives them their orange hue. Just be sure to buy the unsulphured, preservative-free type of apricots instead of the bright-orange, sulfide-treated kind, which can be sensitive to baby.

½ cup (55 g) shredded carrots

¼ cup (33 g) finely diced dried apricots

½ to 1 cup (120 to 235 ml) water

MICROWAVE METHOD: Place the carrots, apricots, and ½ cup (120 ml) water in a 2-cup (475 ml) microwave-safe bowl and microwave on high 5 minutes. Allow to cool slightly and then purée in a blender or mash with a fork until smooth. Add more water if needed to achieve desired consistency.

STOVETOP METHOD: Bring the carrots, apricots, and 1 cup (235 ml) water to a boil in a small saucepan over medium heat. Cover, reduce heat, and simmer 5 to 10 minutes. Allow to cool slightly and then purée in a blender or mash with a fork until smooth. Add more water if needed to achieve desired consistency.

YIELD: 4 baby servings, 2 tablespoons (28 g) each

EACH SERVING CONTAINS: 30.4 calories; 0.1 g total fat; 0.0 grams saturated fat; 0.0 mg cholesterol; 12.0 mg sodium; 7.7 g carbohydrates; 0.5 g dietary fiber; 0.5 g protein; 9.8 mg calcium; 0.5 mg iron; 3615.2 IU vitamin A; and 1.7 mg vitamin C.

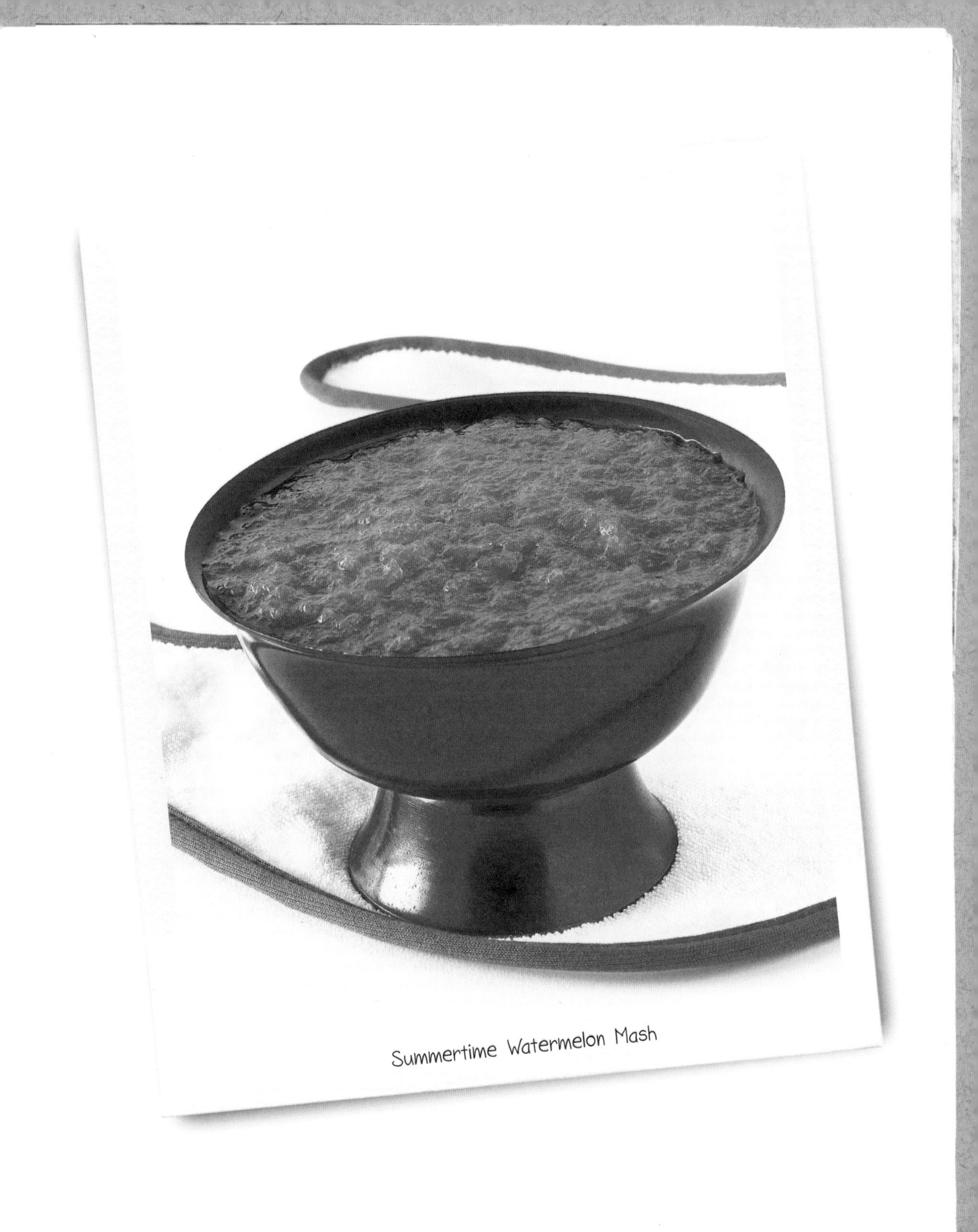

Summertime Watermelon Mash

Blueberry Cottage Cheese with Ease

This is such a simple yet tasty meal for baby. It makes a nice breakfast or snack.

1/4 cup (36 g) blueberries

1/4 cup (55 g) whole milk cottage cheese

1/4 cup (60 ml) breast milk or formula

Wash blueberries. In a blender, combine all ingredients, adding more cottage cheese for a thicker consistency or more breast milk or formula for a thinner consistency.

YIELD: 6 baby servings, 3 tablespoons (45 g) each

EACH SERVING (if using breast milk) CONTAINS: 20.7 calories; 0.9 g total fat; 0.5 grams saturated fat; 3.5 mg cholesterol; 38.5 mg sodium; 2.1 g carbohydrates; 0.2 g dietary fiber; 1.2 g protein; 10.3 mg calcium; 0.0 mg iron; 41.8 IU vitamin A; and 1.1 mg vitamin C.

A-OK Puréed Carrots with Apple

Everyone loves apples. They're versatile, tasty, and healthy. Combined with carrots, they make a nutrient-rich combination that will become your baby's favorite.

1/4 apple

4 baby carrots

2 tablespoons (28 ml) water

MICROWAVE METHOD: Peel, core, and chop apple. Cut the carrots in half lengthwise, then in half again, and place in a small glass bowl with the apple and water. Cover and microwave on high 2 minutes. Allow to cool slightly and then purée in a blender or mash with a fork. Add apple juice, breast milk, or formula if needed to achieve desired consistency.

YIELD: 2 to 4 baby servings, 2 tablespoons (28 g) each

EACH SERVING CONTAINS: 10.6 calories; 0.1 g total fat; 0.0 grams saturated fat; 0.0 mg cholesterol; 11.1 mg sodium; 2.6 g carbohydrates; 0.6 g dietary fiber; 0.2 g protein; 5.8 mg calcium; 0.1 mg iron; 2677.2 IU vitamin A; and 1.3 mg vitamin C.

MOST-EXCELLENT MOUTHFULS:

RECIPES FOR NINE MONTHS

By this age, your little one will be eating three meals daily, and her rapid growth rate will demand more calorie-dense foods. Poultry, beef, and ham can all be introduced now to provide additional sources of nutrition and calories. She also can be encouraged to feed herself and touch her food since this will help her develop the skills she'll need later on to hold a spoon or fork. Just keep in mind that a child will only truly be able to feed herself properly around the age of two or three. Until then, encourage and support her efforts with patience and praise.

Helpful Hints for the High Chair

The following are some reminders and recommendations for preparing food for your nine-month-old:

- Continue feeding 1/2 cup (115 g) single-grain baby rice, barley, or oatmeal cereal, but change to a thicker consistency. You can now also add wheat cereal if there is no allergy to wheat in the family. Serve a vitamin C–rich food such as papaya with the cereal for better iron absorption.
- Serve 1/3 cup (85 g) cooked and mashed or cut up vegetables per day. Use vegetables rich in vitamins A and C such as sweet potatoes and broccoli. (See "All About: Vitamins" on page 192.)
- Offer 1/3 cup (85 g) peeled, cored, and/or seeded ripe fruit per day, either mashed or as finger food.
- Offer one well-cooked egg yolk two to four times a week. Start with 1 tablespoonful (15 g) at a time, adding more if your baby indicates she is still hungry and wants more.

NEW BITES FOR YOUR NINE-MONTH-OLD

Continue to give breast milk or formula to your baby three to four times a day (22 to 32 ounces [650 to 950 ml] total). After nine months, you can make these additions to your baby's diet, in addition to incorporating what baby already enjoys from the previous sections:

VEGETABLES (cooked)	• Broccoli • Cauliflower • Spinach	**DAIRY**	• Yogurt
FRUITS	• Cantaloupe • Papaya	**MEAT**	• Beef • Ham • Poultry
JUICE	• Cantaloupe • Papaya Nectar • Red Grape	**OTHER**	• Soy • Tofu

What to Do When Your Child Refuses Food

When your child exhibits a strong dislike for a certain food, accept it without any fuss. Foods with similar nutritional content can be substituted. Offer the refused food again after a few days and you may find your infant's tastes have changed.

In addition, do not verbally reinforce your child's dislike of a food. Psychologically, this may cause him to resist trying it again at a later time. Also be aware that if family members are fussy eaters, their rejection of many foods may be modeled to the child, so try to keep everyone in a positive state of mind and don't make a big fuss about food rejection. Be patient and try introducing the food again at another time.

When introducing a rejected food for another try—or any food at all—start with a very tiny portion. Your baby may initially look at it, feel it, or just smell it. This is part of the learning process. Some children reject all foods of a certain texture, so it may help to combine a soft food with a chewy food. The color and attractiveness of food influence appetites as well. Mix the colors of vegetables to make them more appealing, for example, by combining small pieces of cauliflower, broccoli, and yellow squash. Most of all, have fun! If you're enjoying the experience, your baby is certain to as well.

Happy Potato with Hard-Cooked Egg Yolk

This is an alternative to plain, hard-cooked egg yolks. A baked or microwaved potato can be substituted for boiled.

1 small unpeeled cooked potato

1 hard-cooked egg yolk

1 to 2 tablespoons (15 to 28 ml) breast milk or formula

1 teaspoon butter (optional)

STOVETOP METHOD: Mash cooked potato with a fork. Mash the cooked egg yolk and combine with potato. Add the breast milk or formula and butter (if desired) and mix well.

YIELD: 3 baby servings, 2 heaping tablespoons (35 to 40 g) each

EACH SERVING (if using breast milk and no butter) CONTAINS: 130.3 calories; 2.2 g total fat; 0.7 grams saturated fat; 73.3 mg cholesterol; 12.5 mg sodium; 24.8 g carbohydrates; 2.3 g dietary fiber; 3.4 g protein; 15.3 mg calcium; 1.4 mg iron; 129.4 IU vitamin A; and 12.5 mg vitamin C.

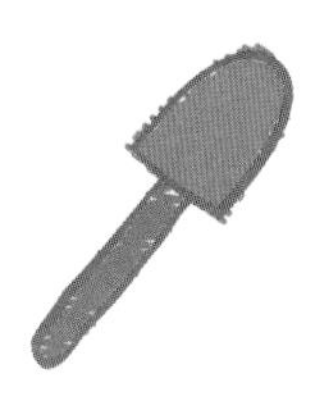

Good Golly Green Beans with Carrot and Apple

Green beans may also be labeled as "string beans" at your market. The vitamin C from the apple in this recipe will increase iron absorption from the green beans for an all-around, well-balanced meal.

1 thinly sliced green bean

1 thinly sliced baby carrot

1 tablespoon to ¼ cup (15 to 60 ml) water

¼ apple

1 to 2 tablespoons (15 to 28 ml) breast milk, formula, or apple juice

MICROWAVE METHOD: Combine the green bean, carrot, and 1 tablespoon (15 ml) water in a small glass bowl. Cover and microwave on high 2 minutes. Peel, core, and cube apple and add it to the dish. Continue cooking 30 seconds. Mash with the breast milk, formula, or apple juice or allow to cool and purée in blender.

STOVETOP METHOD: Peel, core, and cube apple. Place the green bean, carrot, ¼ cup (60 ml) water, and apple cubes in a small pan. Cover and bring to a boil. Reduce the heat and simmer 5 minutes. Mash the mixture with breast milk, formula, or apple juice or allow to cool and purée in blender.

YIELD: 2 baby servings, 2 tablespoons (28 g) each

EACH SERVING (if using breast milk) CONTAINS: 43.0 calories; 0.8 g total fat; 0.3 grams saturated fat; 2.2 mg cholesterol; 6.5 mg sodium; 7.6 g carbohydrates; 1.5 g dietary fiber; 1.8 g protein; 15.7 mg calcium; 0.5 mg iron; 716.7 IU vitamin A; and 2.0 mg vitamin C.

Baby's Favorite Puréed Papaya

Papaya is rich in vitamin C and beta-carotene. Before cutting the papaya, be sure to wash it well. You can even scrub it lightly with a vegetable brush. This is a good habit and sanitary practice to adopt before preparing or eating any fruit.

½ small papaya

¼ cup (60 ml) breast milk or formula

Cut papaya in half and remove the seeds. Scoop the flesh into a blender and add the breast milk or formula. Purée until smooth, scraping down the sides of the blender as necessary.

YIELD: 4 baby servings, 2 tablespoons (28 g) each

EACH SERVING (if using breast milk) CONTAINS: 28.3 calories; 0.7 g total fat; 0.3 grams saturated fat; 2.2 mg cholesterol; 5.1 mg sodium; 5.8 g carbohydrates; 0.5 g dietary fiber; 0.2 g protein; 14.9 mg calcium; 0.1 mg iron; 132.7 IU vitamin A; and 23.3 mg vitamin C.

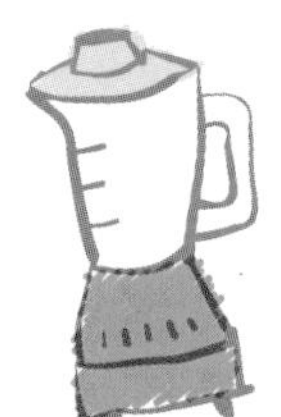

Easy-Peasy Prune and Papaya Purée

Prunes are sometimes referred to as dried plums. This recipe is naturally sweet. What's more, leftovers are the perfect topping for an adult's frozen vanilla yogurt!

8 pitted, dried plums

2 tablespoons (28 ml) prune juice

¼ cup (45 g) diced papaya

Place all ingredients in blender and purée.

YIELD: 3 baby servings, 2 tablespoons (28 g) each

EACH SERVING CONTAINS: 59.8 calories; 0.1 g total fat; 0.0 grams saturated fat; 0.0 mg cholesterol; 3.2 mg sodium; 15.7 g carbohydrates; 2.1 g dietary fiber; 0.5 g protein; 11.4 mg calcium; 8.0 mg iron; 497.4 IU vitamin A; and 8.5 mg vitamin C.

Creamy Broccoli for Baby

Broccoli can sometimes be strong-tasting for babies, so mash it with breast milk or formula. It will mellow the taste and make it more pleasing.

1 broccoli floret

1 tablespoon (15 ml) water (if microwaving)

1 to 2 tablespoons (15 to 28 ml) breast milk, formula, or carrot juice

MICROWAVE METHOD: Place the broccoli in a small microwave-safe bowl with 1 tablespoon (15 ml) water. Cover and microwave on high 1 to 2 minutes until soft. Mash with breast milk, formula, or carrot juice.

STOVETOP METHOD: Place the broccoli in a steamer basket in a saucepan with a little water. Cover and steam over medium-high heat 5 minutes. Mash the broccoli with the breast milk, formula, or carrot juice.

YIELD: 1 baby serving, or 2 tablespoons (28 g)

EACH SERVING (if using 2 tablespoon [28 g] breast milk) CONTAINS: 25.7 calories; 1.4 g total fat; 0.6 grams saturated fat; 4.3 mg cholesterol; 11.5 mg sodium; 2.7 g carbohydrates; 0.8 g dietary fiber; 0.9 g protein; 30.4 mg calcium; 0.4 mg iron; 563.8 IU vitamin A; and 5.4 mg vitamin C.

Incredible Cauliflower Purée

This is a simple, nutritious recipe that can easily be mixed with potato, beans, or just a touch of butter for added flavor and nutrition. Raw cauliflower will keep in the refrigerator for up to one week.

1 (2-inch or 5 cm) cauliflower floret

1 tablespoon (15 ml) water

1 tablespoon (15 ml) breast milk, formula, or carrot juice

MICROWAVE METHOD: Place the cauliflower in a small microwave-safe bowl with water. Cover and microwave on high 1 to 2 minutes or until soft. Mash with the breast milk, formula, or carrot juice.

STOVETOP METHOD: Place the cauliflower in a steamer basket in a saucepan with a little water; cover and steam over medium-high heat 5 minutes. Mash the cauliflower with the breast milk, formula, or carrot juice.

YIELD: 1 baby serving, or 2 tablespoons (28 g)

EACH SERVING (if using breast milk) CONTAINS: 14.9 calories; 0.8 g total fat; 0.3 grams saturated fat; 2.2 mg cholesterol; 5.3 mg sodium; 1.8 g carbohydrates; 0.4 g dietary fiber; 0.5 g protein; 7.8 mg calcium; 0.1 mg iron; 34.8 IU vitamin A; and 8.7 mg vitamin C.

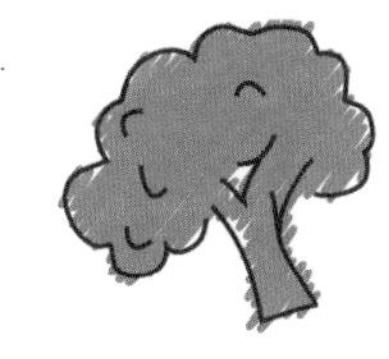

Little Bunny's Favorite Cauliflower and Carrot

Both cauliflower and carrots are inexpensive and very healthy, making this meal cost-effective for you and nutritious for your baby.

1 baby carrot

1 (2-inch or 5 cm) cauliflower floret

¼ cup (60 ml) water

1 teaspoon unsalted butter

MICROWAVE METHOD: Slice the carrot into small pieces. Combine the carrot, cauliflower, and water in a small glass bowl. Cover and microwave on high 3 minutes. Purée or mash with the butter or serve as finger food.

YIELD: 1 baby serving, or 3 tablespoons (45 g)

EACH SERVING CONTAINS: 43.1 calories; 3.7 g total fat; 2.7 grams saturated fat; 10 mg cholesterol; 14.9 mg sodium; 2.2 g carbohydrates; 0.8 g dietary fiber; 0.4 g protein; 8.1 mg calcium; 0.1 mg iron; 2808.0 IU vitamin A; and 7.0 mg vitamin C.

Sweet Omelet Surprise

Different variations of this recipe are simple to make. Just replace the apple with ¼ cup (55 g) mashed papaya, plum, banana, or grated or mashed pear.

¼ cup (55 g) apple

1 teaspoon unsalted butter

2 egg yolks

1 tablespoon (15 ml) water, formula, or breast milk

STOVETOP METHOD: Peel, core, and chop the apple. Heat the butter in a small frying pan over low heat. Add the apple and cook for 1 minute. In a small bowl, whisk the egg yolks with the water, formula, or breast milk and pour over the apples. Cook, turning once, until the egg is well set. Cool and cut into small strips or pieces and serve as finger food.

YIELD: 4 baby servings, 2 tablespoons (28 g) each

EACH SERVING (if using breast milk) CONTAINS: 43.1 calories; 3.4 g total fat; 1.6 grams saturated fat; 108.0 mg cholesterol; 4.8 mg sodium; 2.0 g carbohydrates; 0.2 g dietary fiber; 1.4 g protein; 12.8 mg calcium; 0.3 mg iron; 169.5 IU vitamin A; and 0.7 mg vitamin C.

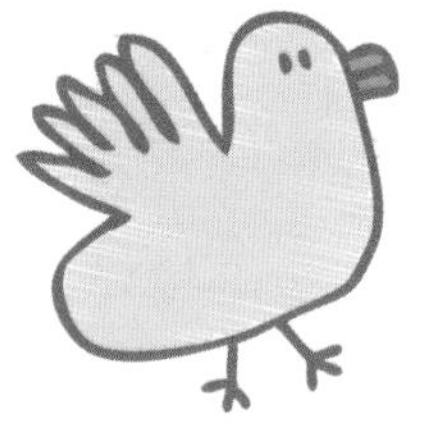

Egg-cellent Fried Rice

Babies love rice—and we all love fried rice! To make this recipe, use a mild-flavored oil such as canola or corn.

2 tablespoons (28 g) cooked brown rice

1 egg yolk

1 teaspoon vegetable oil

STOVETOP METHOD: Mix the cooked rice and egg yolk in a cup. Heat the oil in a small frying pan over medium heat. Add the rice mixture and mold into a small pancake with a spatula. Cook well on one side, turn, and continue to cook until well done. Cool and cut into pieces and serve as finger food.

YIELD: 2 baby servings, 2 tablespoons (28 g) each

EACH SERVING CONTAINS: 56.5 calories; 4.1 g total fat; 2.2 grams saturated fat; 109.9 mg cholesterol; 4.2 mg sodium; 3.1 g carbohydrates; 0.0 g dietary fiber; 1.6 g protein; 12.0 mg calcium; 0.4 mg iron; 189.2 IU vitamin A; and 0.0 mg vitamin C.

Yummy in My Tummy Banana-Yogurt Puddin'

Yogurt is a good source of protein and includes other important nutrients, including calcium, potassium, vitamin B-12, and magnesium.

1 teaspoon unsalted butter

2 to 4 tablespoons (28 to 56 g) mashed banana

1 to 2 tablespoons (15 to 30 g) plain yogurt

STOVETOP METHOD: Melt the butter in a frying pan over low heat. Combine banana and yogurt and add the mixture to the pan. Stir well until heated through. Cool and serve.

YIELD: 3 baby servings, 2 tablespoons (28 g) each

EACH SERVING (using 2 tablespoons [28 g] banana and 1 tablespoon [15 g] yogurt) CONTAINS: 34.5 calories; 1.3 g total fat; 0.9 grams saturated fat; 3.5 mg cholesterol; 6.0 mg sodium; 5.6 g carbohydrates; 0.5 g dietary fiber; 0.5 g protein; 11.3 mg calcium; 0.1 mg iron; 56.4 IU vitamin A; and 1.6 mg vitamin C.

Practice Egg Safety!

Fresh eggs may contain salmonella bacteria that can cause an intestinal infection. Healthy adults usually recover in less than a week, but the infection can be very dangerous for infants and toddlers. Eggs should be cooked until both yolk (and white, when baby is ready to eat it) are firm. Scrambled eggs, casseroles, and other dishes containing eggs should be cooked to 160°F (70°C). Use a food thermometer to check the temperature. Serve cooked egg dishes immediately after cooking or refrigerate at once for serving later. Use the dish within three to four days, or freeze for longer storage.

Triple-Tasty Avocado, Cantaloupe, and Yogurt

Any avocado you have remaining from this recipe can be used for an adult lunch or salad, and the rest of the cantaloupe can be used for dessert!

1 slice (½-inch or 12 mm) ripe avocado

1 small slice (¼ inch, or 6 mm) ripe cantaloupe

2 tablespoons (30 g) plain yogurt

Remove any peel from the avocado and cantaloupe and mash together. Serve with the yogurt on the side or mixed in.

YIELD: 2 baby servings, 2½ tablespoons (35 g) each

EACH SERVING CONTAINS: 53.2 calories; 2.1 g total fat; 0.3 grams saturated fat; 0.6 mg cholesterol; 23.8 mg sodium; 7.7 g carbohydrates; 1.2 g dietary fiber; 1.5 g protein; 37.2 mg calcium; 0.2 mg iron; 1078.5 IU vitamin A; and 11.6 mg vitamin C.

Avocado and Peach Mash with Papaya Nectar

Nectar is very thick because it contains fruit pulp. It can be found in both bottles and cans in the "International" or "Ethnic" sections of most supermarkets and in health food stores. Be sure to buy nectars without added sugar, corn syrup, or other additives and preservatives.

¼ small, ripe peach

2 tablespoons (28 g) ripe avocado

1 tablespoon (15 ml) papaya nectar

Peel and cut peach into small pieces. Place the avocado and peach in a small cup and mash lightly. Pour the papaya nectar over the fruit and mix well.

YIELD: 2 baby servings, 2 tablespoons (28 g) each

EACH SERVING CONTAINS: 78.4 calories; 4.6 g total fat; 0.6 grams saturated fat; 0.0 mg cholesterol; 2.7 mg sodium; 10.0 g carbohydrates; 2.8 g dietary fiber; 1.1 g protein; 8.7 mg calcium; 0.3 mg iron; 227.1 IU vitamin A; and 8.6 mg vitamin C.

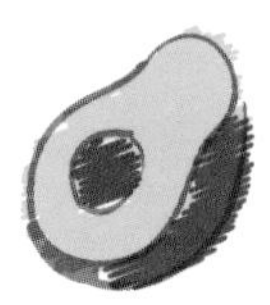

Avocados: A Superfood for All!

Many pediatricians agree that avocado is an ideal first food. It's mild and smooth in taste and is high in healthy monounsaturated fats your baby needs at this age. It also contains iron, vitamin A, folate, and vitamin B6—but no cholesterol.

To easily peel and pit an avocado, cut it in half and twist to separate the two halves. Slip a spoon between the pit and avocado to remove the pit. Then slip the spoon between the skin and the avocado to loosen it. If you like, cut the flesh into slices or cubes before you take it out of the skin.

Yummy Yummy Carrot-Papaya Yogurt

The flesh of the papaya is golden yellow-orange, juicy, and silky smooth, with a sweet and mellow flavor. Be sure to thoroughly remove all the seeds before cooking.

¼ to ½ cup (60 to 120 ml) water

½ cup (55 g) shredded carrots

¼ cup (45 g) peeled, seeded, finely diced ripe papaya

1 tablespoon (15 g) plain yogurt

MICROWAVE METHOD: Place ¼ cup (60 ml) water and the carrots in a microwave-safe glass bowl. Cover and cook on high 4 minutes. Allow to cool slightly and then transfer to a blender. Add the papaya and process 45 seconds. Remove the purée from the blender. Use 1 tablespoon (15 g) of the purée and blend with yogurt. The remaining purée can be stored in the refrigerator for up to 2 days.

STOVETOP METHOD: Combine ½ cup (120 ml) water and the carrots in a small saucepan over medium high heat. Cover and bring to a boil. Allow to cool slightly and then transfer to a blender. Add the papaya and process 45 seconds. Remove the purée from the blender. Use 1 tablespoon (15 g) of the purée and blend with yogurt. The remaining purée can be stored in the refrigerator for up to 2 days.

YIELD: 4 baby servings, 2 tablespoons (28 g) each

EACH SERVING CONTAINS: 11.1 calories; 0.1 g total fat; 0.1 grams saturated fat; 0.2 mg cholesterol; 11.7 mg sodium; 2.4 g carbohydrates; 0.5 g dietary fiber; 0.3 g protein; 11.3 mg calcium; 0.1 mg iron; 2392.8 IU vitamin A; and 6.2 mg vitamin C.

Lucky Peas, Lucky Me!

A thicker purée can be achieved by reducing the amount of breast milk or formula. A pinch of mild curry powder is a great addition after your baby is one year old.

¼ cup (33 g) frozen peas

1 heaping tablespoon (15 to 20 g) plain yogurt

¼ cup (60 ml) breast milk or formula

MICROWAVE METHOD: Cook and drain frozen peas according to package instructions. Mix together all ingredients in a microwave-safe bowl. Microwave 10 to 15 seconds until warm. Mash with a fork and serve.

YIELD: 2 baby servings, 2 tablespoons (28 g) each

EACH SERVING (if using breast milk) CONTAINS: 42.0 calories; 1.7 g total fat; 0.9 grams saturated fat; 5.8 mg cholesterol; 10.6 mg sodium; 5.0 g carbohydrates; 0.8 g dietary fiber; 1.5 g protein; 24.4 mg calcium; 0.3 mg iron; 152.5 IU vitamin A; and 2.7 mg vitamin C.

Yummy Recipe Tip: Use Whatever's On Hand

You can substitute the same amount of ripe, fresh apricots or plums for the papaya in the yogurt recipe at left.

Baby's First Chicken with Corn and Potatoes ❄

Never offer your baby pieces of meat until she has several teeth—and then carefully chop the meat into extra-small, bite-size pieces. This recipe is a wonderful way to introduce your baby to the flavor of chicken.

1 small skinless, boneless chicken breast or chicken tender

¼ cup (53 g) canned corn

1 small white potato

Cook and dice chicken. Drain canned corn. Peel, boil, and dice potato. Put all ingredients into a blender and pulverize until smooth. Push mixture through a sieve to remove any lumps or skin from the corn. Add a touch of breast milk or formula if desired to get a creamy consistency.

YIELD: 4 baby servings, 3 tablespoons (45 g) each

EACH SERVING CONTAINS: 81.7 calories; 2.0 g total fat; 0.5 grams saturated fat; 6.4 mg cholesterol; 109.5 mg sodium; 12.1 g carbohydrates; 1.1 g dietary fiber; 3.5 g protein; 7.6 mg calcium; 0.6 mg iron; 3.7 IU vitamin A; and 3.9 mg vitamin C.

Lovely Little Pasta Soup

Pastina literally means "little pasta," and is commonly used in soups. This recipe will easily adapt to your baby's age and tastes. Try adding Bright Eyes Mashed Carrots (page 58), Dreamy Creamy Spinach (page 83), or tiny bits of broccoli, chicken, or turkey.

1½ cups (355 ml) low-sodium chicken broth

2 (22 g) tablespoons uncooked pastina

STOVETOP METHOD: Bring broth to a gentle boil and add pastina. Cook, stirring frequently, 7 or 8 minutes or until pastina is cooked. Serve warm.

This recipe, covered tightly, will last for 2 to 3 days in the refrigerator. To reheat, just add a bit of water.

YIELD: 4 baby servings, ¼ cup (55 g) each

EACH SERVING CONTAINS: 50.8 calories; 0.2 g total fat; 0.1 grams saturated fat; 1.9 mg cholesterol; 225.6 mg sodium; 9.6 g carbohydrates; 0.4 g dietary fiber; 2.4 g protein; 2.2 mg calcium; 0.4 mg iron; 0.5 IU vitamin A; and 0.0 mg vitamin C.

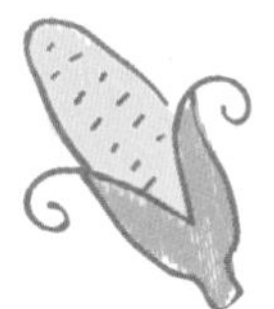

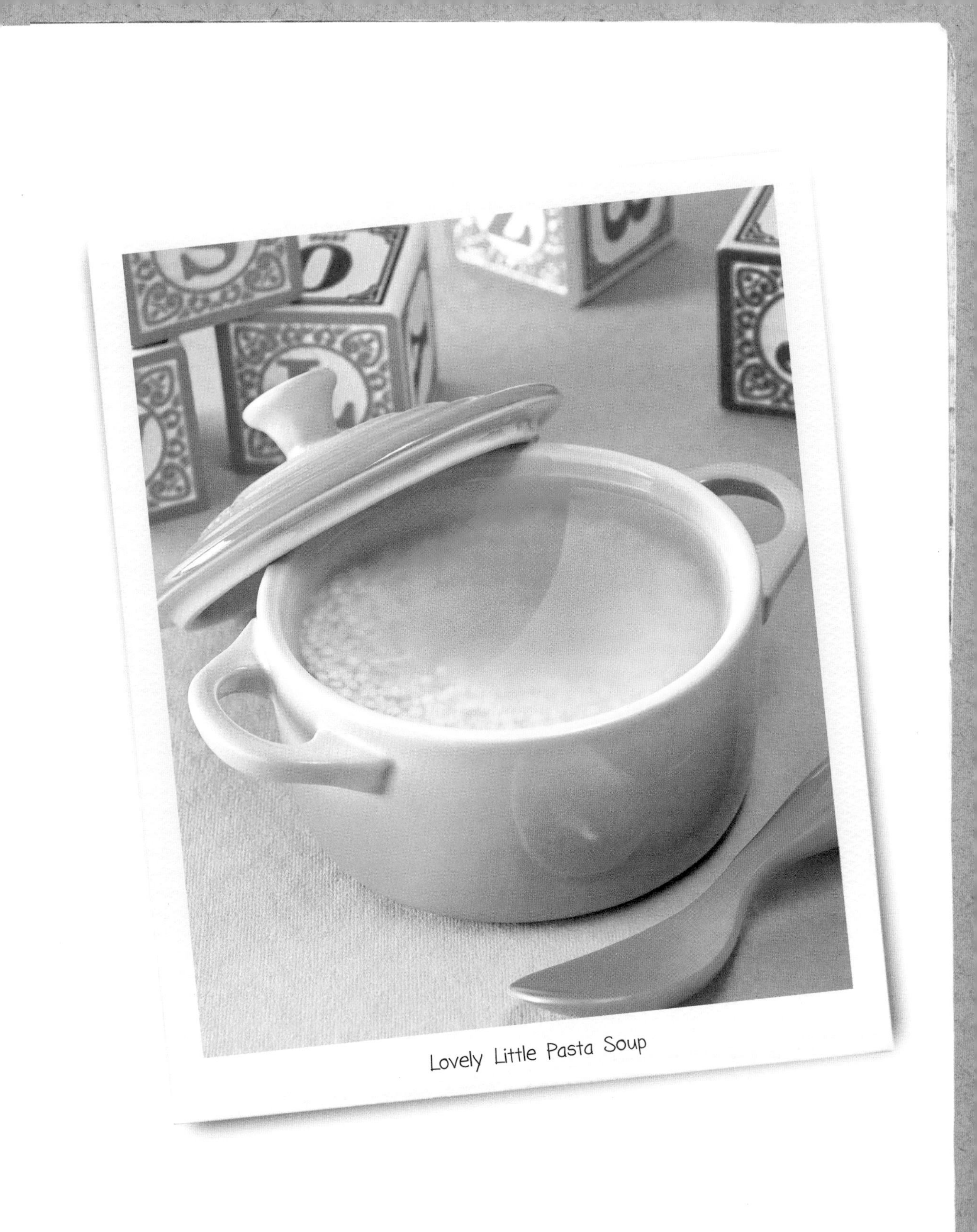

Lovely Little Pasta Soup

Chicken with Sweet Potatoes ❄

Chicken purée has a better texture when blended with a root vegetable. If you don't have sweet potatoes on hand, the flesh of a white potato will produce similar results.

1 small skinless, boneless chicken breast or chicken tender

1 small sweet potato

Cook and dice chicken. Peel, boil, and dice potato. Put all ingredients into a blender and pulverize until smooth. Add a touch of breast milk or formula if desired to get a creamy consistency.

This recipe, covered tightly, will last 2 to 3 days in the refrigerator.

YIELD: 6 baby servings, 1/4 cup (55 g) each

EACH SERVING CONTAINS: 33.4 calories; 1.2 g total fat; 0.3 grams saturated fat; 4.3 mg cholesterol; 45.5 mg sodium; 3.9 g carbohydrates; 0.3 g dietary fiber; 1.7 g protein; 4.7 mg calcium; 0.2 mg iron; 1980.6 IU vitamin A; and 1.6 mg vitamin C.

Practice Poultry Safety!

When buying fresh chicken or turkey, the package should feel cold and have a sell-by date of several days beyond the purchase date. Make the grocery store your last stop before going home. Once home, immediately put the chicken in a refrigerator that maintains a temperature of 40°F (4°C). Use the poultry within 1 or 2 days or freeze at 0°F (-18°C). Whole chicken and ground chicken and turkey can be frozen up to one month, if well wrapped.

Follow instructions on the package about how to handle the chicken during preparation. For safety, tenderness, and doneness, cook a whole chicken to 180°F (82°C). Use a food thermometer and insert it into the thigh or thickest part of the meat.

When making poultry dishes using ground chicken or turkey, be sure the meat is thoroughly cooked, with no red or pink showing. A meat thermometer should register at 170°F (77°C).

Highchair Haute Chicken with Peaches

As your baby becomes used to "solid" food, you can make this purée a bit chunkier to encourage chewing. This recipe is also delicious with Naturally Sweet Apricot Purée (page 56).

1 small skinless, boneless chicken breast or chicken tender

2 tablespoons (28 g) Fuzzy Peach Purée (page 48)

Cook and dice chicken. Put all ingredients into a blender and pulverize until smooth. Add a touch of breast milk or formula if desired to get a creamy consistency.

YIELD: 4 baby servings, 2 tablespoons (28 g) each

EACH SERVING CONTAINS: 44.4 calories; 2.5 g total fat; 0.5 grams saturated fat; 6.2 mg cholesterol; 64.8 mg sodium; 3.1 g carbohydrates; 0.3 g dietary fiber; 2.3 g protein; 2.6 mg calcium; 0.2 mg iron; 14.5 IU vitamin A; and 0.4 mg vitamin C.

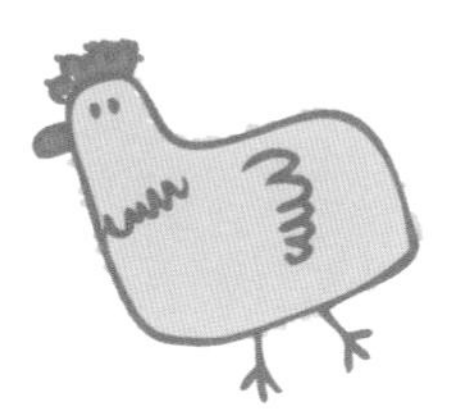

Dreamy Creamy Spinach

You can use chopped, frozen spinach in this recipe to save time. And don't forget to always use unsalted butter!

½ cup (80 g) thawed, drained, and chopped frozen spinach

1 tablespoon (14 g) unsalted butter

¼ cup (60 ml) breast milk or formula

Place all contents in blender and purée until creamy.

This recipe, covered tightly, will last 2 days in the refrigerator.

YIELD: 4 baby servings, 2 tablespoons (28 g) each

EACH SERVING (if using breast milk) CONTAINS: 47.1 calories; 3.4 g total fat; 2.3 grams saturated fat; 9.7 mg cholesterol; 50.0 mg sodium; 2.2 g carbohydrates; 0.4 g dietary fiber; 0.9 g protein; 35.2 mg calcium; 0.3 mg iron; 1079.6 IU vitamin A; and 1.2 mg vitamin C.

Broccoli Au Gratin

Broccoli is a nutrient-dense vegetable. One cup (71 g) of broccoli provides as much vitamin C as an orange, and it's also a good source of fiber and folate.

1 cup (71 g) small broccoli florets

¼ cup (60 ml) water

¼ cup (30 g) grated mild Cheddar cheese

1 tablespoon (7 g) plain breadcrumbs

MICROWAVE METHOD: Microwave broccoli in water for 2 minutes or until soft. Add cheese. Mash with fork and sprinkle with breadcrumbs.

YIELD: 4 baby servings, 2 tablespoons (28 g) each

EACH SERVING CONTAINS: 26.9 calories; 0.5 g total fat; 0.3 grams saturated fat; 1.3 mg cholesterol; 73.8 mg sodium; 2.5 g carbohydrates; 0.8 g dietary fiber; 2.5 g protein; 32.5 mg calcium; 0.1 mg iron; 50.0 IU vitamin A; and 7.5 mg vitamin C.

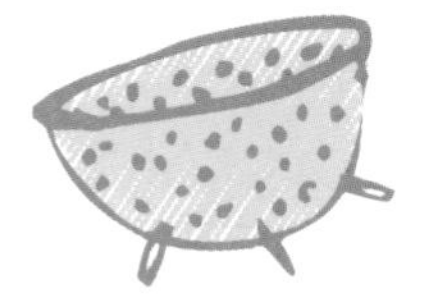

Chicken in the Grass

Try making this recipe with the dark meat of the chicken. It has more than twice the iron as the white meat.

1 small skinless, boneless chicken breast or chicken tender

¼ cup (55 g) Dreamy Creamy Spinach (page 83)

MICROWAVE METHOD: Cook and dice chicken. In a small microwave-safe bowl, warm the chicken and spinach for 15 seconds. Mash together. If you'd like, serve with steamed couscous on the side or mixed in.

YIELD: 6 baby servings, 2 tablespoons (28 g) each

EACH SERVING CONTAINS: 36.0 calories; 2.3 g total fat; 0.5 grams saturated fat; 5.8 mg cholesterol; 77.4 mg sodium; 2.1 g carbohydrates; 0.5 g dietary fiber; 1.8 g protein; 14.2 mg calcium; 0.3 mg iron; 16.7 IU vitamin A; and 0.8 mg vitamin C.

Sweet Potato and Cauliflower Purée

A baby's eating habits are naturally erratic, so keep in mind your goal is simply to introduce your baby to new flavors and textures. Recipes in this book can be easily scaled up or down for that reason—in many cases, like this one, the ratio is a simple 1:1 for ingredients.

1 tablespoon (15 g) Oh So Sweet Potato Purée (page 34)

1 tablespoon (15 g) Incredible Cauliflower Purée (page 75)

Mash together ingredients and serve. Add a touch of breast milk or formula if desired to get a creamy consistency.

YIELD: 1 baby serving, or 2 tablespoons (28 g)

EACH SERVING CONTAINS: 23.0 calories; 0.8 g total fat; 0.4 grams saturated fat; 2.5 mg cholesterol; 10.2 mg sodium; 3.5 g carbohydrates; 0.5 g dietary fiber; 0.5 g protein; 8.9 mg calcium; 0.1 mg iron; 539.2 IU vitamin A; and 6.4 mg vitamin C.

Summertime Puréed Banana with Papaya

This is a quick and easy no-cook recipe that's packed with nutrition. Remember, for best results, make no-cook purées just before you're ready to serve them.

½ small, ripe banana

¼ small, ripe papaya (about ¼ cup, or 35 g)

Mash together the banana and papaya flesh and serve.

YIELD: 4 baby servings, 2 tablespoons (28 g) each

EACH SERVING CONTAINS: 21.9 calories; 0.1 g total fat; 0.0 grams saturated fat; 0.0 mg cholesterol; 1.4 mg sodium; 5.4 g carbohydrates; 0.6 g dietary fiber; 0.2 g protein; 5.7 mg calcium; 0.1 mg iron; 5.9 IU vitamin A; and 12.5 mg vitamin C.

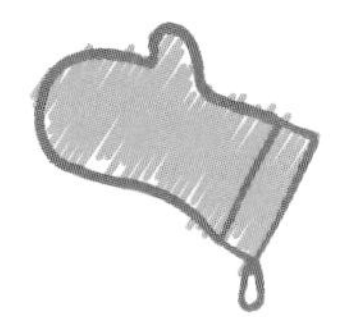

It's a Bird! It's a Plane! It's Super Papaya!

Papaya is an excellent source of potassium and vitamins A and C. It also contains a protein-digesting enzyme that is used as a remedy for indigestion.

Naturally Nutritious Cantaloupe and Pear Purée

Cantaloupe is a rich source of vitamins A and C, while pears are a good source of both copper and fiber. Just keep in mind that puréed melon doesn't freeze well, so use this recipe within a day or two.

1 slice (1⁄4-inch or 6 mm) ripe cantaloupe

2 tablespoons (28 ml) pear nectar

1 tablespoon (15 g) Sweet Pear Purée (page 29)

Blend the cantaloupe in a blender with the pear nectar. Combine cantaloupe mixture with Sweet Pear Purée and serve.

YIELD: 4 baby servings, 2 tablespoons (28 g) each

EACH SERVING CONTAINS: 70.6 calories; 0.2 g total fat; 0.1 grams saturated fat; 0.0 mg cholesterol; 17.9 mg sodium; 17.8 g carbohydrates; 2.0 g dietary fiber; 1.0 g protein; 13.4 mg calcium; 0.4 mg iron; 3456.8 IU vitamin A; and 47.1 mg vitamin C.

Any Way You Please Chicken with Peas ❄

You can easily adjust the consistency of this recipe by modifying the size of the chopped chicken. If you'd prefer the consistency of a purée, whip together both ingredients in a blender.

1 small skinless, boneless chicken tender

2 tablespoons (28 g) Lucky Peas, Lucky Me! (page 79)

Cook and finely dice chicken. Combine with peas and serve warm.

YIELD: 4 baby servings, 1 tablespoon (15 g) each

EACH SERVING CONTAINS: 46.8 calories; 2.7 g total fat; 0.6 grams saturated fat; 7.0 mg cholesterol; 66.1 mg sodium; 3.0 g carbohydrates; 0.3 g dietary fiber; 2.4 g protein; 5.6 mg calcium; 0.2 mg iron; 19.1 IU vitamin A; and 0.3 mg vitamin C.

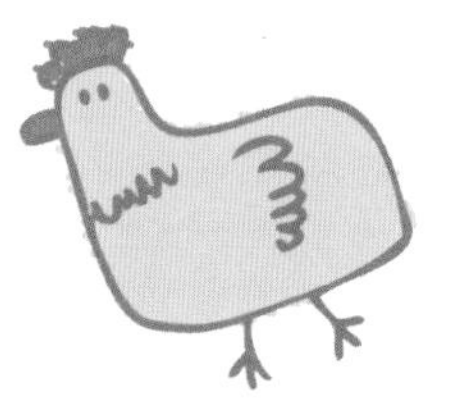

Tropical Chicken and Papaya Purée

This purée makes a nice lunch or dinner option for baby. Frozen chicken tenders should be a pantry staple. They cook within 15 minutes, and they're just the right size for a baby.

1 small skinless, boneless chicken tender

2 tablespoons (28 g) Summertime Puréed Banana with Papaya (page 85)

Cook and finely dice chicken. Combine ingredients in a blender and serve warm.

YIELD: 4 baby servings, 1 tablespoon (15 g) each

EACH SERVING CONTAINS: 45.1 calories; 2.6 g total fat; 0.6 grams saturated fat; 6.5 mg cholesterol; 65.4 mg sodium; 3.1 g carbohydrates; 0.3 g dietary fiber; 2.3 g protein; 4.4 mg calcium; 0.2 mg iron; 16.6 IU vitamin A; and 2.9 mg vitamin C.

Growing Strong Beef and Potato Purée ❄

At this age, babies become less satisfied with the standard menu of grains, fruit, and vegetables, so beef can provide a nourishing, high-protein meal. Beef is also an excellent source of iron.

2 ounces (55 g) cooked ground beef (do not add salt or oil)

2 tablespoons (28 g) Oh So Sweet Potato Purée (page 34)

1/4 cup (60 ml) breast milk or formula

Place all ingredients in a blender. Purée, adding breast milk or formula to achieve desired consistency.

YIELD: 4 baby servings, 2 tablespoons (28 g) each

EACH SERVING (if using breast milk) CONTAINS: 60.6 calories; 3.6 g total fat; 1.5 grams saturated fat; 15.7 mg cholesterol; 18.8 mg sodium; 2.8 g carbohydrates; 0.2 g dietary fiber; 4.0 g protein; 12.5 mg calcium; 0.4 mg iron; 383.2 IU vitamin A; and 2.1 mg vitamin C.

Start Slow with Meat

Meat has a very different taste and texture than what your baby has become used to, so it's normal that infants are slow to adopt meat protein. Begin with one tablespoon (15 g) servings. If your baby accepts this serving size, increase the portion according to his appetite.

Beef and Carrot Purée

If your baby makes a funny face when he tries this for the first time, don't stop feeding him the food completely. He might be reacting to the new texture, not the flavor.

2 ounces (55 g) cooked ground beef (do not add salt or oil)

1 tablespoon (15 ml) low-sodium beef or chicken broth

2 tablespoons (28 g) Bright Eyes Mashed Carrots (page 58)

2 teaspoons plain yogurt

Combine all ingredients in a blender and purée to desired consistency. Microwave purée for 10 to 15 seconds or until warm.

YIELD: 4 baby servings, 2 tablespoons (28 g) each

EACH SERVING CONTAINS: 43.6 calories; 2.8 g total fat; 1.2 grams saturated fat; 13.4 mg cholesterol; 27.7 mg sodium; 0.6 g carbohydrates; 0.1 g dietary fiber; 3.8 g protein; 7.4 mg calcium; 0.4 mg iron; 168.3 IU vitamin A; and 0.0 mg vitamin C.

Creamy Turkey and Spinach

This recipe can be assembled quickly using leftovers. If you don't have cooked turkey, skinless, boneless cooked chicken or leftover ground beef will work nicely too.

2 ounces (55 g) cooked turkey

2 tablespoons (28 g) Dreamy Creamy Spinach (page 83)

2 tablespoons (28 ml) breast milk or formula

Dice cooked turkey. Combine with other ingredients in a blender. Serve warm.

YIELD: 4 baby servings, 2 tablespoons (28 g) each

EACH SERVING (if using breast milk) CONTAINS: 52.0 calories; 3.2 g total fat; 1.3 grams saturated fat; 18.3 mg cholesterol; 30.5 mg sodium; 1.2 g carbohydrates; 0.1 g dietary fiber; 4.2 g protein; 15.9 mg calcium; 0.4 mg iron; 320.3 IU vitamin A; and 0.7 mg vitamin C.

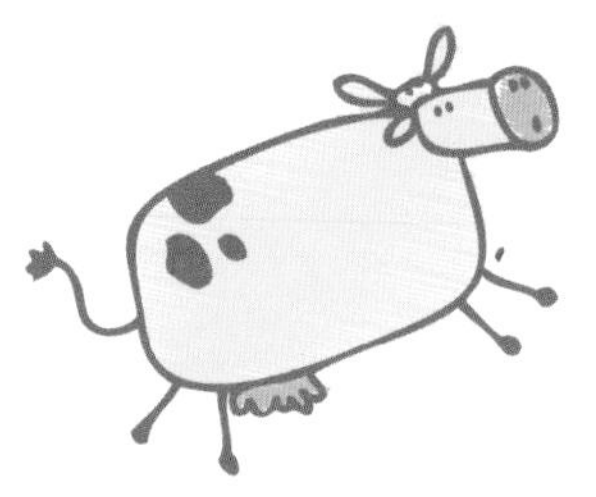

NATURALLY NOURISHING BITES:

RECIPES FOR TEN MONTHS

At ten months of age, your baby's diet will start to resemble the rest of the family's. She will eat three to four small meals a day and continue to make progress in self-feeding, but she may not be able to use a spoon independently until after her first birthday. Until then, fill the spoon and help her guide it to her mouth. Talk to your baby while feeding her, and tell her the name and the colors of the food on her plate. She's sure to love it (and you)!

Helpful Hints for the High Chair

Here are some useful tips to keep in mind for feeding time:

- Always strap your baby in a high chair while he is eating and watch your baby the whole time he is eating and drinking. As babies grow, they develop an amazing ability to wiggle out of high chairs.
- The intake from one meal to the next may vary dramatically. Over the course of a day, your baby will eat what he needs. Make sure he can choose from a variety of wholesome foods.
- Encourage your baby to drink from a cup to help develop coordination and foster independence.
- Each day, offer up to ⅓ cup (85 g) fruit and ⅓ cup (85 g) peeled soft-cooked vegetables rich in vitamins A, B, and C, such as carrots, beans, and kiwi. (See "All About: Vitamins" on page 192.)
- Offer 1 to 4 tablespoons (15 to 55 g) of legumes such as split peas or lentils per day.
- Offer 1 to 4 tablespoons (15 to 55 g) of rice or noodles per day.

NEW BITES FOR YOUR TEN-MONTH-OLD

While you should continue feeding your baby breast milk or formula, three to four times a day (20 to 32 ounces [570 to 950 ml] total), at ten months, you can make these additions to your baby's diet:

VEGETABLES (cooked)	• Bell Peppers • Cabbage • Celery • Leek • Parsley • Parsnip
FRUITS	• Cherries (halved and pitted) • Kiwi • Melons
JUICE	• Blueberry • Cherry • Kiwi
DAIRY (whote fat)	• Cream cheese • Jack cheese • Mozzarella (fresh or soft) • Swiss cheese
GRAINS	• Crackers • Pasta • Whole wheat breads
LEGUMES	• Lentils • Split peas
OTHER	• Pancakes • Waffles

Scrambling for More Egg and Cheese

The egg is a nutrition powerhouse. One egg has thirteen essential nutrients, most of which are in the yolk. Remember that babies this age are not supposed to eat egg whites, only the yolks.

1 teaspoon oil or butter

1 egg yolk

1 tablespoon (15 ml) breast milk, formula, or water

1 tablespoon (7 g) grated Swiss cheese

STOVETOP METHOD: Heat the oil in a small frying pan over medium heat. In a bowl, whisk together the egg yolk; breast milk, formula, or water; and cheese. Pour into the frying pan and stir until cooked through completely. Cut into thin strips or pieces and serve warm.

YIELD: 1 baby serving, or 1/4 cup (55 g)

EACH SERVING CONTAINS: 125.5 calories; 10.9 g total fat; 5.7 grams saturated fat; 228.2 mg cholesterol; 25.8 mg sodium; 1.9 g carbohydrates; 0.0 g dietary fiber; 4.6 g protein; 101.9 mg calcium; 0.5 mg iron; 486.1 IU vitamin A; and 0.8 mg vitamin C.

Gotta Love 'em Lentils

Carrots, celery, and potatoes may also be cooked together with the lentils and mashed. Leftover cooked lentils can be frozen in small batches.

1/2 cup (100 g) cooked brown lentils

Cook lentils according to package directions. Mash with a fork and add unsalted butter if desired.

YIELD: 2 baby servings, 1/4 cup (55 g) each

EACH SERVING CONTAINS: 57.4 calories; 0.2 g total fat; 0.0 grams saturated fat; 0.0 mg cholesterol; 1.0 mg sodium; 10.0 g carbohydrates; 4.0 g dietary fiber; 4.5 g protein; 9.4 mg calcium; 1.7 mg iron; 4.0 IU vitamin A; and 0.7 mg vitamin C.

Yummy Recipe Tip: Lend a New Flavor to Your Lentils

For a new twist, serve lentils with cooked carrots, celery, rice, potatoes, bananas, avocados, or puréed apricots.

Lentil and Banana Mash

Brown lentils are mild tasting, and if you overcook them and they get mushy, don't worry. The softer the lentils are, the better they work when making baby food. You can also try red or green lentils if your baby doesn't like the flavor of the brown variety.

2 tablespoons (25 g) cooked brown lentils

2 tablespoons (28 g) mashed ripe banana

Cook lentils according to package directions. Mash the lentils and banana together. Warm gently over low heat, if desired.

YIELD: 1 baby serving, or 1/4 cup (55 g)

EACH SERVING CONTAINS: 53.7 calories; 0.2 g total fat; 0.0 grams saturated fat; 0.0 mg cholesterol; 0.8 mg sodium; 11.4 g carbohydrates; 2.7 g dietary fiber; 2.5 g protein; 6.1 mg calcium; 0.9 mg iron; 20.0 IU vitamin A; and 2.8 mg vitamin C.

Cook Up a Pot, Use It All Week!

To save time when making meals that call for lentils, split peas, or other dry beans, cook one-quarter of a pound (about 1/2 cup, or 95 g dry) and keep them in the refrigerator until you're ready to use them. They'll last three to four days in a tightly sealed container. If your baby doesn't finish what you've made, use them yourself! Whip them up in a food processor for a nutritious lentil hummus spread or put them in green salads, sandwiches, or wraps.

Crib-Rockin' Lentil Roast ❄

This dish is also tasty with just lentils, sweet potato, and carrots mashed together with butter (hold the eggs and juice).

1 teaspoon oil or butter

1/4 cup (50 g) cooked brown lentils

1/4 sweet potato, peeled, cooked, and mashed

3 baby carrots, cooked and mashed

1 tablespoon (14 g) unsalted butter

2 egg yolks, beaten

1/4 cup (60 ml) apple juice

OVEN METHOD: Preheat the oven to 350°F (180°C, gas mark 4). Grease a small ovenproof dish with oil or butter. In a small bowl, mix together the prepared lentils, potato, carrots, and butter. In another bowl, whisk the egg yolks and apple juice. Blend with the lentil mix. Pour into the baking dish, cover, and bake in a water bath 30 to 45 minutes. (A water bath is just a roasting pan that has been filled with 1 1/2 to 2 inches [38 to 50 mm] of water. The hot water provides a constant heat source and ensures even cooking. Place your baking dish into the water-filled roasting pan and then put the pan into the oven.) Let cool before serving. Divide any unused leftovers into small portions and freeze.

YIELD: 4 baby servings, 1/4 cup (55 g) each

EACH SERVING CONTAINS: 82.1 calories; 4.2 g total fat; 2.3 grams saturated fat; 109.9 mg cholesterol; 34.2 mg sodium; 8.5 g carbohydrates; 1.4 g dietary fiber; 2.8 g protein; 27.4 mg calcium; 0.9 mg iron; 2372.5 IU vitamin A; and 5.6 mg vitamin C.

Naturally Nutritious Lentil Mash ❄

Lentils are a legume, or bean, and they're an inexpensive source of protein. While not all beans are the same in terms of protein quality, lentils are among the best for baby to enjoy.

½ cup (100 g) cooked brown lentils

1 small potato, peeled, cubed and cooked

4 baby carrots, sliced and cooked

1 small stalk celery, sliced and cooked

1 tablespoon (14 g) unsalted butter, softened

Place the prepared lentils, potato, carrots, and celery in a bowl. Add the butter and mash with a fork. Divide the leftovers into small portions and freeze, if you wish. Serve lukewarm.

YIELD: 4 baby servings, ¼ cup (55 g) each

EACH SERVING CONTAINS: 81.3 calories; 2.7 g total fat; 2.0 grams saturated fat; 7.5 mg cholesterol; 18.5 mg sodium; 11.5 g carbohydrates; 2.2 g dietary fiber; 2.3 g protein; 14.4 mg calcium; 0.8 mg iron; 937.8 IU vitamin A; and 5.9 mg vitamin C.

Finger-Lickin' Good Lentils with Potato and Cheese

This recipe also works well with mild Cheddar, Jarlsberg, or Edam cheeses. Jarlsberg is also called "Baby Swiss," and Edam is a bit like Gouda.

2 tablespoons (25 g) cooked lentils

1 small cooked potato

1 tablespoon (7 g) grated Swiss cheese

MICROWAVE METHOD: Mash the cooked lentils and potato and mix together. Place in a microwave-safe dish and sprinkle with the cheese. Microwave on medium until warmed through, less than 60 seconds. Cool, stir, and check food temperature before serving.

YIELD: 2 baby servings, ¼ cup (55 g) each

EACH SERVING CONTAINS: 97.0 calories; 1.3 g total fat; 0.7 grams saturated fat; 3.6 mg cholesterol; 3.6 mg sodium; 17.4 g carbohydrates; 2.6 g dietary fiber; 4.1 g protein; 57.6 mg calcium; 1.2 mg iron; 50.8 IU vitamin A; and 9.1 mg vitamin C.

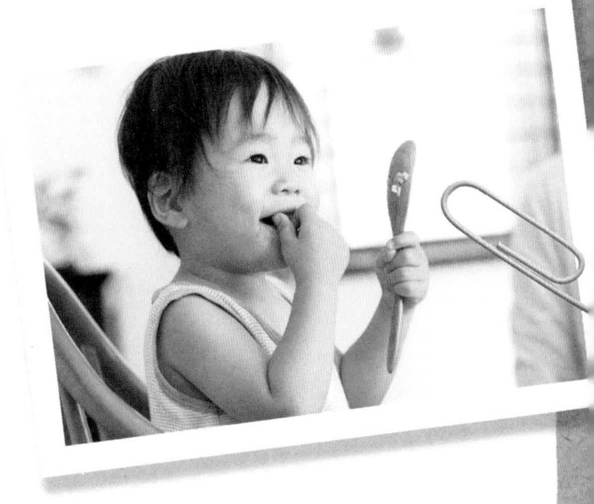

Dreamy Green Beans

Green beans are a rich source of protein, fiber, and complex carbohydrates. They're also called string beans or snap beans, so be on the lookout for all three guises.

4 green beans

2 tablespoons (28 ml) water

1 tablespoon (15 g) plain yogurt

1 tablespoon (15 g) cream cheese

MICROWAVE METHOD: Trim, quarter, and cook the green beans. Place all ingredients into a blender and liquefy. Warm in microwave for 15 seconds or serve at room temperature.

YIELD: 2 baby servings, 2 tablespoons (28 g) each

EACH SERVING CONTAINS: 37.8 calories; 2.7 g total fat; 1.6 grams saturated fat; 9.0 mg cholesterol; 30.1 mg sodium; 2.0 g carbohydrates; 0.7 g dietary fiber; 1.0 g protein; 23.0 mg calcium; 23.0 mg iron; 166.0 IU vitamin A; and 0.4 mg vitamin C.

Wahooo! Split Pea Stew ❄

Split peas are just the dried version of the modern-day garden pea, cut in half. They are a good source of fiber, protein, folate, and potassium.

1 small cooked potato

1 small cooked carrot

½ cup (55 g) cooked split green peas

Peel and cube the cooked potato. Peel and chop the cooked carrot. Mash the cooked split green peas, potato, and carrot and add butter, if desired. Divide any leftover stew into small portions and freeze.

YIELD: 3 baby servings, ¼ cup (55 g) each

EACH SERVING CONTAINS: 95.9 calories; 0.2 g total fat; 0.0 grams saturated fat; 0.0 mg cholesterol; 13.2 mg sodium; 20.3 g carbohydrates; 4.0 g dietary fiber; 3.9 g protein; 11.8 mg calcium; 0.7 mg iron; 2614.0 IU vitamin A; and 8.5 mg vitamin C.

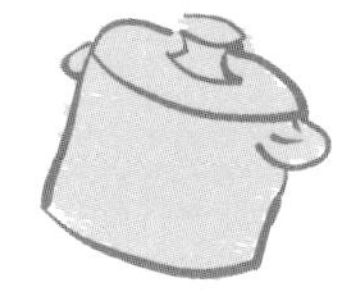

A Dozen Healthy Finger Foods

Running out of ideas for healthy bites your baby can enjoy? Try some of these:

- Cooked noodles or macaroni
- Cooked sweet potato chunks (or other vegetables)
- Crackers or graham crackers
- Fresh grated carrots and apples
- Grilled cheese on toast cut into small quarters
- Lightly cooked apple wedges
- Pancakes or waffles
- Small pieces of cooked tofu
- Soft avocado pieces
- Toast with butter or mashed bananas
- Unsweetened dry cereal without nuts, honey, or dried fruit
- Wedges of soft, ripe fruit

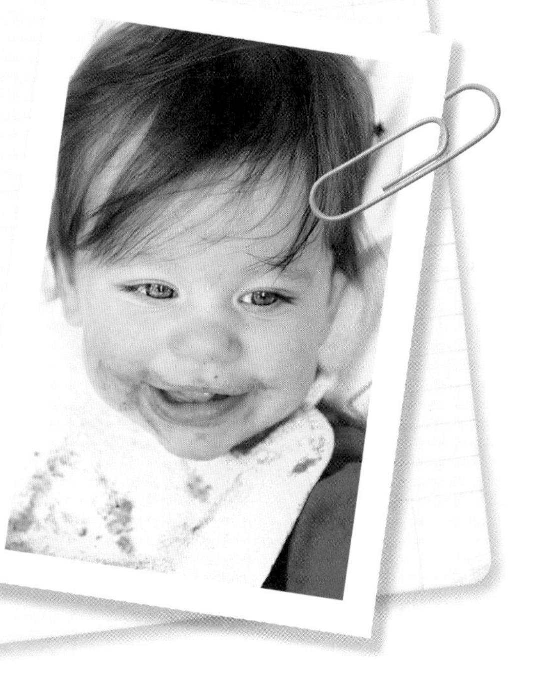

Creamy Apricot Parfait

For a thinner result, add a bit more fruit purée to this recipe. Use less purée if you want a thicker consistency. If you mix all of the ingredients together, you can use this recipe as a spread on toast, bagels, waffles, crackers, or even mixed into brown rice!

1 tablespoon (15 g) cream cheese

1 tablespoon (15 g) plain yogurt

1 tablespoon (15 g) Naturally Sweet Apricot Purée (page 56)

Mix the cream cheese and yogurt well with a fork and top with the apricot purée.

YIELD: 1 baby serving, or 3 tablespoons (45 g)

EACH SERVING CONTAINS: 67.4 calories; 5.5 g total fat; 3.1 grams saturated fat; 18.0 mg cholesterol; 54.0 mg sodium; 3.2 g carbohydrates; 0.2 g dietary fiber; 1.5 g protein; 34.3 mg calcium; 0.2 mg iron; 390.9 IU vitamin A; and 0.1 mg vitamin C.

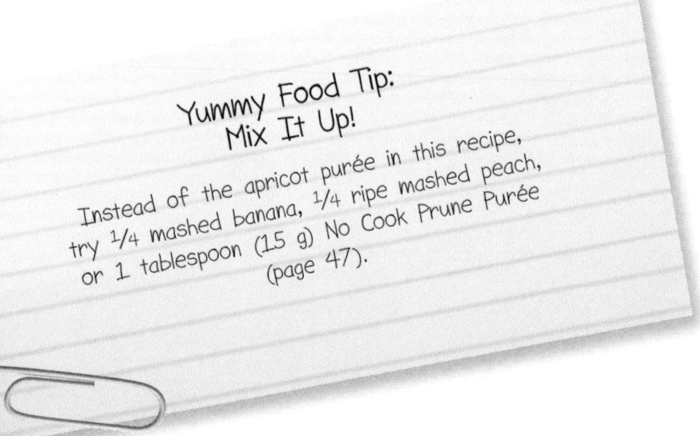

Steamed Cauliflower with Swiss

This recipe is pure comfort food. Experiment with different cheeses to find your baby's favorite.

3 cauliflower florets

1 tablespoon (15 ml) water

1 tablespoon (8 g) shredded Swiss cheese

MICROWAVE METHOD: Place the cauliflower in a small glass bowl with the water. Cover and microwave on high 1 to 2 minutes or until soft. Transfer to a plate, let cool slightly, and cut into small pieces or mash lightly. Sprinkle with the cheese.

STOVETOP METHOD: Place the cauliflower in a steamer basket with water and steam 5 minutes or until soft. Transfer to a plate, let cool slightly, and cut into small pieces or mash lightly. Sprinkle with the cheese.

YIELD: 1 baby serving, or 3 tablespoons (45 g)

EACH SERVING CONTAINS: 40.0 calories; 2.2 g total fat; 1.2 grams saturated fat; 6.3 mg cholesterol; 23.1 mg sodium; 2.5 g carbohydrates; 1.2 g dietary fiber; 3.0 g protein; 83.7 mg calcium; 0.2 mg iron; 81.5 IU vitamin A; and 23.9 mg vitamin C.

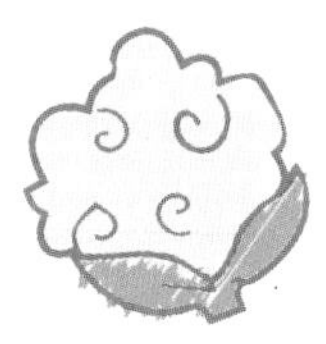

Tofu, Cheese, and Scrambled Egg Yolks

Tofu is low in saturated fats and has no cholesterol, preservatives, coloring, or additives. Silken tofu will last five to seven days in the refrigerator.

2 tablespoons (30 g) silken tofu

2 egg yolks

1 tablespoon (15 ml) water

½ teaspoon unsalted butter

2 tablespoons (16 g) shredded Cheddar, provolone, or any other cheese on hand

STOVETOP METHOD: Place the tofu, egg yolks, and water in a blender and process for 3 seconds. Melt the butter in a small frying pan over medium heat. Pour the tofu-egg mix into the frying pan. Stir in the cheese and scramble until the mixture is cooked through.

YIELD: 2 baby servings, 3 tablespoons (45 g) each

EACH SERVING (if using Cheddar) CONTAINS: 81.3 calories; 6.1 g total fat; 2.5 grams saturated fat; 213.5 mg cholesterol; 63.2 mg sodium; 1.0 g carbohydrates; 0.3 g dietary fiber; 5.4 g protein; 56.8 mg calcium; 0.6 mg iron; 328.5 IU vitamin A; and 0.0 mg vitamin C.

Top-Notch Tofu and Apricot Purée

Tofu is a protein-rich food made from the curds of soybean milk. It's also a good source of both iron and manganese. This purée is delicious served with cooked brown rice or Basmati rice.

¼ cup (60 g) silken tofu

¼ cup (55 g) Naturally Sweet Apricot Purée (page 56)

Place the tofu and Naturally Sweet Apricot Purée in a blender and process until smooth.

YIELD: 2 baby servings, ¼ cup (55 g) each

EACH SERVING CONTAINS: 45.6 calories; 0.6 g total fat; 0.0 grams saturated fat; 0.0 mg cholesterol; 1.5 mg sodium; 7.6 g carbohydrates; 0.6 g dietary fiber; 1.5 g protein; 24.0 mg calcium; 0.7 mg iron; 726.9 IU vitamin A; and 0.0 mg vitamin C.

Tofu: What's It All About?

Tofu, one of the more common soy products, is rich in protein and contains all eight essential amino acids. A good source of calcium (when fortified), tofu also supplies sufficient amounts of choline and vitamin E. It is soft, very easily digested, and an excellent food for babies.

Like yogurt or cottage cheese, tofu is ready to eat and requires no preparation. It's versatile and can be steamed, microwaved, broiled, sautéed, toasted, or baked. Tofu can also be sliced, cubed, mashed, puréed, frozen, dried, or blended. To store tofu, place it in a clean container with some fresh water and store it in the refrigerator. If the water is changed every day, it will keep for a week. Silken, soft tofu does not come in water. Follow the directions on the package for how to store it.

Hand-in-Hand Cabbage and Apple

Cabbage and apple go together like cookies and milk. Gala, Fuji, and Rome apples will all work well in this recipe, but feel free to use whatever you have or find available.

1 apple

1 cup (70 g) finely shredded cabbage

1⁄3 cup (80 ml) water

STOVETOP METHOD: Peel, core, and cut apple into wedges. Place the apple, cabbage, and water in a small saucepan over medium heat. Slowly bring to a simmer, cover, and cook 5 minutes until the cabbage and apple are soft. Add more water, if needed. Lightly mash and add butter if desired.

YIELD: 4 baby servings, 1⁄4 cup (55 g) each

EACH SERVING CONTAINS: 30.6 calories; 0.1 g total fat; 0.0 grams saturated fat; 0.0 mg cholesterol; 6.5 mg sodium; 7.9 g carbohydrates; 1.6 g dietary fiber; 0.4 g protein; 12.7 mg calcium; 0.2 mg iron; 272.9 IU vitamin A; and 14.8 mg vitamin C.

Cabbage: Good for Baby Budget

Cabbage (both red and Savoy) is high in calcium, vitamin C, and folate. Buy the smallest cabbage you can find—a one-pound (455 g) head of cabbage—goes a long way! Remaining cabbage can be used in adult coleslaw, stir-fries, and soups.

Five Little Finger Sandwiches

Little sandwiches make the perfect meal or snack. Plus, they don't require cooking, just "assembly."

Here are some favorite combos:

Cream cheese and jam

Mashed banana and maple syrup

Grated carrot and cream cheese

Shredded cheese and mashed avocado

Refried beans and mashed avocado

Choose filling and assemble. Remove the crust from the bread, cut the sandwich into small pieces, or cut out with cookie cutters.

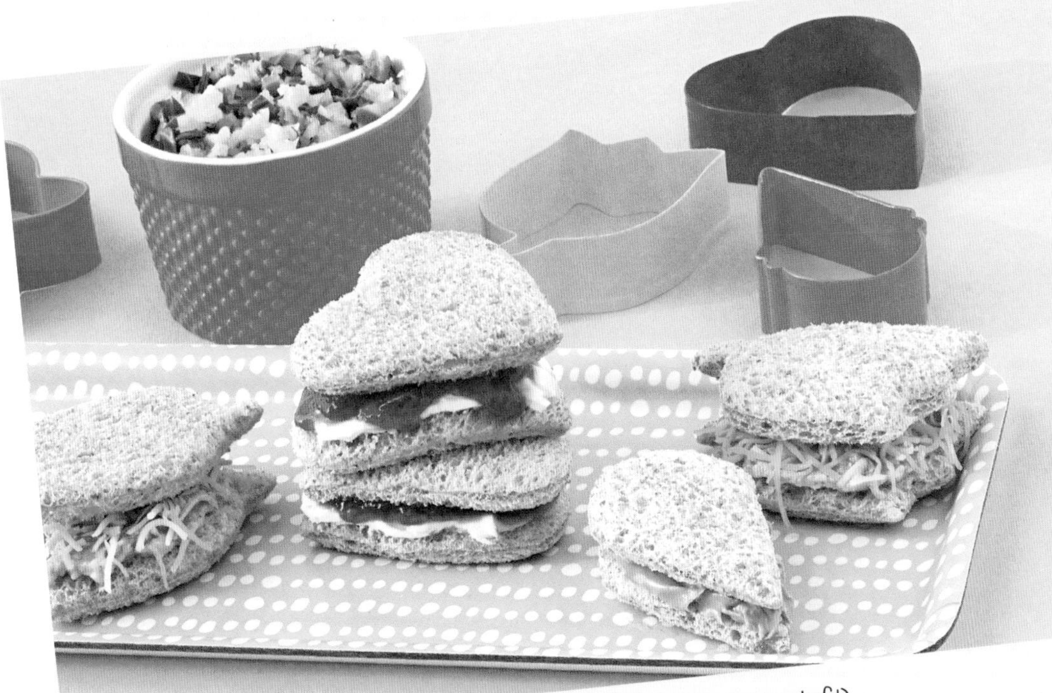

Hand-in-Hand Cabbage and Apple (top left)
and Five Little Finger Sandwiches (foreground)

Bubble and Squeak

Bubble and Squeak is a traditional English meal. With the exception of coleslaw and corned beef and cabbage on St. Patrick's Day, cabbage is not too popular in America, but it's a shame! It makes a healthy and delicious meal for baby and a great side dish for the whole family. Be sure to finely grate the cabbage for best results.

2 small red potatoes

1⁄4 leek

1⁄2 cup (35 g) finely grated cabbage

3⁄4 cup (175 ml) water

2 tablespoons (28 g) unsalted butter

STOVETOP METHOD: Peel and dice potatoes. Wash and finely chop the leak. Place the potato, cabbage, leek, and water in a medium saucepan over medium-high heat. Bring to a boil, reduce the heat, cover, and simmer 20 minutes; add water if needed. When the potato and cabbage are soft and the water is almost absorbed, add the butter and mash.

YIELD: 5 baby servings, 1⁄4 cup (55 g) each

EACH SERVING CONTAINS: 90.6 calories; 4.5 g total fat; 3.2 grams saturated fat; 12.0 mg cholesterol; 6.5 mg sodium; 11.5 g carbohydrates; 1.4 g dietary fiber; 1.4 g protein; 11.2 mg calcium; 0.6 mg iron; 281.6 IU vitamin A; and 11.2 mg vitamin C.

Red Light, Green Light Bell Pepper and Beans

This brightly colored dish is one your baby will love. Talk about colors when you feed her.

6 green beans

1⁄4 small red bell pepper

STOVETOP METHOD: Cut beans and pepper into thin strips, making sure to remove any seeds from the pepper. Place the vegetables in a steamer basket and steam until soft. Cool and serve as finger food.

YIELD: 2 baby servings, 1⁄4 cup (55 g) each

EACH SERVING CONTAINS: 52.1 calories; 0.2 g total fat; 0.1 grams saturated fat; 0.0 mg cholesterol; 2.5 mg sodium; 9.4 g carbohydrates; 2.5 g dietary fiber; 3.5 g protein; 19.4 mg calcium; 1.0 mg iron; 305.8 IU vitamin A; and 12.5 mg vitamin C.

Roasting Red Bell Peppers

All bell peppers are good sources of vitamin C, but red bell peppers have twice as much vitamin C as green peppers. For your baby, purée roasted peppers with a little breast milk or formula for a delicious meal. Here's a quick how-to:

1. Preheat the broiler. In the meantime, wash the peppers and cut in half (do not remove stems and seeds).
2. Place peppers, cut side down, on a baking sheet covered with a piece of tinfoil, 3 inches (7.5 cm) below the broiler. Broil until the halves are blackened.
3. Carefully remove and place peppers in a sealed plastic bag for 15 minutes. Remove the skin, stems, and seeds (they should slip off easily) and cut into strips or purée. Use any leftovers on pizza or in pasta or sandwiches.

Veggies with Tofu

This meal can be poured into baby's sippy cup if he'd prefer to drink his veggies. Just make sure all ingredients are whipped into a smooth liquid.

1/4 cup (56 g) peeled and diced sweet potato

3 small carrots, peeled and diced

2 tablespoons (28 ml) water

1 tablespoon (14 g) unsalted butter

1/4 cup (60 ml) breast milk or formula

1/4 cup (60 g) silken tofu

MICROWAVE METHOD: Place sweet potatoes and carrots in a microwave safe bowl with water. Cover and microwave for 2 minutes. Transfer vegetables and liquid to blender with butter and breast milk or formula. Cut tofu into small pieces and add. Liquefy, let cool, and serve.

YIELD: 3 baby servings, 1/4 cup (55 g) each

EACH SERVING (if using breast milk) CONTAINS: 69.8 calories; 5.0 g total fat; 3.1 grams saturated fat; 12.9 mg cholesterol; 11.9 mg sodium; 4.6 g carbohydrates; 0.5 g dietary fiber; 1.3 g protein; 24.5 mg calcium; 0.2 mg iron; 3391.5 IU vitamin A; and 3.6 mg vitamin C.

Sweet Apple "Cream"

This is a sweet and natural dessert for your little one. If you don't have apple juice concentrate, try orange juice concentrate for an orange "cream."

1/4 cup (60 g) cream cheese

2 tablespoons (36 g) frozen apple juice concentrate

Place the cheese and juice concentrate into blender and whip until creamy.

YIELD: 1 baby serving

EACH SERVING CONTAINS: 258.4 calories; 19.8 g total fat; 11.2 grams saturated fat; 63.8 mg cholesterol; 186.2 mg sodium; 16.7 g carbohydrates; 0.0 g dietary fiber; 3.4 g protein; 56.8 mg calcium; 0.2 mg iron; 733.3 IU vitamin A; and 0.0 mg vitamin C.

Tofu Banana Extravaganza

Tofu is a canvas for just about any ingredient. Experiment with different fruit and tofu combinations to see what your baby likes best.

4 ounces (120 g) firm tofu

1/2 ripe banana

Purée all ingredients in a blender until a fluffy texture is achieved. Serve by spoon or spread on toast for toddlers.

YIELD: 2 baby servings, 1/4 cup (55 g) each

EACH SERVING CONTAINS: 57.7 calories; 1.3 g total fat; 0.7 grams saturated fat; 3.3 mg cholesterol; 14.9 mg sodium; 3.3 g carbohydrates; 1.2 g dietary fiber; 1.6 g protein; 84.6 mg calcium; 3.7 mg iron; 64.6 IU vitamin A; and 35.6 mg vitamin C.

Wee One's Kiwi

Kiwi does not need to be cooked, and it should not need to be seeded. It is typically introduced to baby at an age when she can manage a bit of texture.

1 ripe kiwi

1/4 cup (55 g) Mighty Mouthful Rice Cereal or prepared iron-fortified rice cereal

Peel ripe kiwi. Purée or mash with a fork and add cereal to thicken and achieve a smooth yet thin consistency.

YIELD: 2 baby servings, 1/4 cup (55 g) each

EACH SERVING (using Mighty Mouthful Rice Cereal) CONTAINS: 57.7 calories; 1.3 g total fat; 0.7 grams saturated fat; 3.3 mg cholesterol; 14.9 mg sodium; 10.6 g carbohydrates; 1.2 g dietary fiber; 1.6 g protein; 84.6 mg calcium; 3.8 mg iron; 64.6 IU vitamin A; and 35.6 mg vitamin C.

The Skinny on Soy Products

Protein-rich soy foods are also good sources of iron, calcium, and zinc, making them a staple of many vegetarian diets. Here's how to make sense of some common soy products:

- Tofu: Soy bean curd, made by adding nigari (evaporated seawater) to soy milk, similar to the curd-making process of cheese
- Silken tofu: More finely textured than regular tofu
- Soy nut butter: A spread made from roasted, ground soy beans, similar to peanut butter
- Soy oil: Cooking oil made from pressed soy beans
- Tempeh: A cake made from fermented soy beans with a nutty flavor and firm texture
- Miso: Fermented soy bean paste, dissolved in water as a base for soups (lighter miso is less strongly flavored than darker varieties.)
- Textured vegetable protein (TVP): Made from soy bean flour and used as a meat substitute

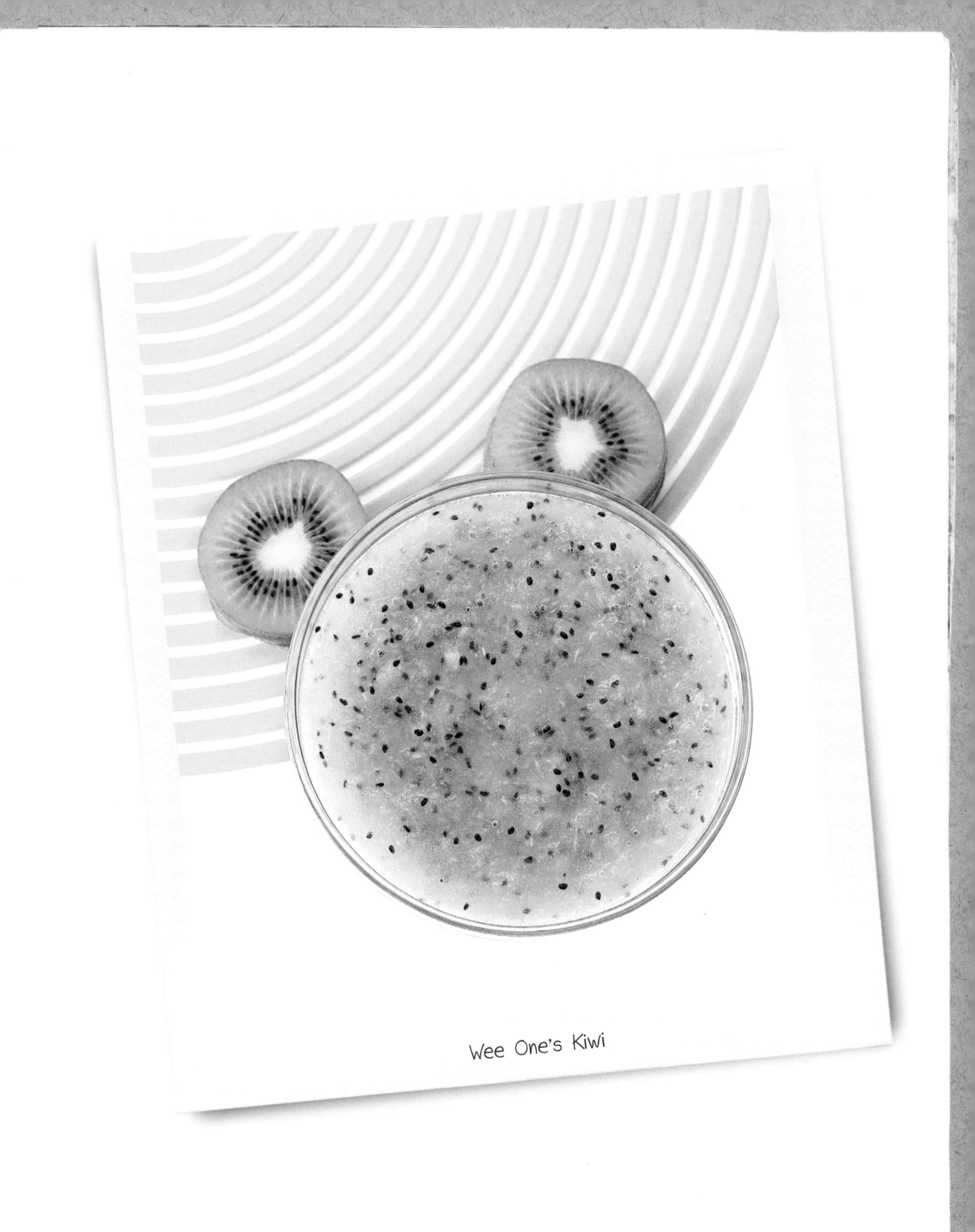

Wee One's Kiwi

Ham and Cheese Pastina, Please

Meat has a very different texture than fruit or vegetables, so be patient when feeding baby new proteins. Eventually, your little one will except them.

1 ounce (28 g) cooked ham

1/4 cup (44 g) cooked pastina

2 tablespoons (14 g) shredded cheese such as mozzarella or Swiss

MICROWAVE METHOD: Finely dice the ham. Combine ham, pastina, and cheese in a microwave-safe dish. Cook on high for 30 seconds. Remove from microwave and stir until cheese is melted. Serve lukewarm.

YIELD: 4 baby servings, 2 tablespoons (28 g) each

EACH SERVING CONTAINS: 73.5 calories; 1.3 g total fat; 0.7 grams saturated fat; 5.3 mg cholesterol; 943.8 mg sodium; 11.7 g carbohydrates; 0.5 g dietary fiber; 3.7 g protein; 22.9 mg calcium; 0.5 mg iron; 27.0 IU vitamin A; and 0.0 mg vitamin C.

Ga-Ga Graham Crackers and Yogurt

This recipe strikes the perfect balance between flavor and texture. Cinnamon graham crackers are a nice alternative to plain.

2 unsweetened graham crackers

2 tablespoons (30 g) plain yogurt

2 tablespoons (28 g) mashed banana

Finely crumble the graham crackers in a small bowl. Add the yogurt and mashed banana. Mix together and serve.

YIELD: 2 baby servings, 3 tablespoons (45 g) each

EACH SERVING CONTAINS: 57.1 calories; 0.9 g total fat; 0.2 grams saturated fat; 1.3 mg cholesterol; 49.1 mg sodium; 11.5 g carbohydrates; 0.6 g dietary fiber; 1.1 g protein; 14.9 mg calcium; 0.3 mg iron; 9.1 IU vitamin A; and 1.2 mg vitamin C.

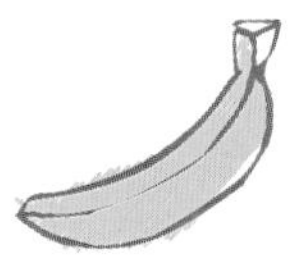

Make Your Own Yogurt Cheese—It's Easy!

Yogurt cheese is plain yogurt that has been drained of its whey so its texture resembles cream cheese. To make yogurt cheese, line a colander with several layers of clean cheesecloth (or use a yogurt drainer, a small sieve with a muslin liner). Fill the colander with pasteurized whole-milk yogurt. Place the colander in a container that will catch the whey, leaving at least 1 1/2 inches (3.5 cm) for the liquid to drain off. Cover and refrigerate 8 to 12 hours. Use the cheese as a substitute for sour cream or cream cheese. And don't throw out the whey! It can be added to soups, stews, or smoothies.

WHOLESOME MEALS FOR A HAPPY HEAD START:

RECIPES FOR ELEVEN MONTHS

At eleven months of age, your baby is nearly a toddler, and he might start getting a bit fussy about what's on his plate. But picky eaters tend to try things that their friends are eating, so when the going gets rough, call your mommy friends, have them bring their little ones over for lunch, and serve some new recipes from this section. Your child might see the other children enjoying the lunch you prepared and begin cleaning his plate, too!

Helpful Hints for the High Chair

Here are some useful tips to keep in mind for feeding time. Do the following each day:

- Offer two to four servings of cereal, whole-grain breads, muffins, crackers, rice (preferably brown), cooked grains, or pasta. Each serving should be about 1⁄4 of an adult serving, such as: 1⁄4 piece of bread, 1⁄4 small muffin, 1⁄4 cup (55 g) cooked or cold cereal, or 1⁄4 cup (55 g) cooked rice or pasta.
- Give three servings of 1 to 2 tablespoons (15 to 28 g) each of fruits and vegetables. Vary the fruits and vegetables introduced during the past five months, so your baby will get all the necessary vitamins. (See "All About: Vitamins" on page 192 and "All About: Minerals" on page 195.)
- In addition to breast milk or formula, serve yogurt, cottage cheese, cream cheese, and ricotta (2 to 4 tablespoons [30 to 60 g], or other cheeses (1⁄2 to 3⁄4 ounces [15 to 22 g]).
- Give two servings (2 ounces [55 g total]) of protein, such as egg yolk, tofu, poultry, beans, and legumes. (See "All About: Proteins" on page 186.)

NEW BITES FOR YOUR ELEVEN-MONTH-OLD

As your baby approaches his eleventh month, most of his nutrition should be coming from solids, and at this time, your little one has been exposed to a variety of foods and knows what he likes and dislikes. At eleven months, you can make these additions to your baby's diet:

BABY CEREAL (cooked)	• Barley • Cream of rice • Cream of wheat • Multi-grain • Oatmeal
VEGETABLES (cooked)	• Beets • Brussels sprouts • Kale • Romaine lettuce (raw) • Rutabaga • Turnips
FRUITS	• Figs • Grapes (seeded and halved) • Pineapple • Raisins (cooked) • Raspberries
DAIRY (whole fat)	• Cheddar cheese • Goat cheese • Parmesan cheese • Romano cheese • Ricotta cheese
LEGUMES	• Black, white, and red beans • Lima beans • Refried beans
OTHER	• Couscous • Polenta

White Beans with Dreamy Creamy Spinach

The smooth texture of white beans goes perfectly with homemade creamed spinach, and together, they provide lots of calcium and vitamin A for baby.

¼ cup (45 g) cooked white beans (homemade or canned and unsalted)

¼ cup (55 g) Dreamy Creamy Spinach (page 83)

Mash beans with a fork. Add creamed spinach and mix well. Warm in microwave and serve.

This recipe, covered tightly, will last for 1 to 2 days in the refrigerator.

YIELD: 2 baby servings, ¼ cup (55 g) each

EACH SERVING CONTAINS: 72.1 calories; 3.7 g total fat; 2.3 grams saturated fat; 9.7 mg cholesterol; 60.0 mg sodium; 6.5 g carbohydrates; 1.6 g dietary fiber; 2.4 g protein; 45.0 mg calcium; 0.7 mg iron; 1079.7 IU vitamin A; and 1.2 mg vitamin C.

Baby's Favorite Broccoli and Beans

Preparing dried beans can take a long time, so don't be afraid to just open a can of beans if you're crunched for time. They are just as nutritious as their dried counterparts.

2 tablespoons (23 g) cooked white beans (homemade or canned and unsalted)

1 small broccoli floret, steamed

1 teaspoon unsalted butter

STOVETOP METHOD: Gently warm the beans in a small saucepan over low heat, adding some of the cooking liquid from the beans if necessary. Add the broccoli and butter and mash with a fork.

This recipe, covered tightly, will last for 1 to 2 days in the refrigerator.

YIELD: 1 baby serving, or 3 tablespoons (about 45 g)

EACH SERVING CONTAINS: 60.2 calories; 4.0 g total fat; 2.7 grams saturated fat; 10.0 mg cholesterol; 11.3 mg sodium; 1.6 g carbohydrates; 1.4 g dietary fiber; 1.6 g protein; 11.0 mg calcium; 0.4 mg iron; 133.3 IU vitamin A; and 1.9 mg vitamin C.

Recipe Variation Tip

For a new twist on this recipe, try mashing the beans with 2 tablespoons (28 g) cooked and mashed carrots, potatoes, sweet potatoes, zucchini, other squash, or avocados.

Black Beans, Avocado, and Yogurt, Oh My!

This is a yummy combination served warm or cold. If the skins of the beans separate in the blender, pour the mixture through a strainer and discard the skins that remain.

¼ cup (43 g) black beans (homemade or canned)

¼ avocado

¼ cup (60 g) plain yogurt

2 teaspoons vegetable oil

Place all ingredients into a blender and purée.

YIELD: 2 baby servings, ¼ cup (55 to 60 g) each

EACH SERVING CONTAINS: 109.7 calories; 7.8 g total fat; 1.8 grams saturated fat; 4.2 mg cholesterol; 25.6 mg sodium; 7.6 g carbohydrates; 2.7 g dietary fiber; 3.4 g protein; 58.4 mg calcium; 0.5 mg iron; 71.1 IU vitamin A; and 1.8 mg vitamin C.

Black Beans and Rice, Sounds Nice

Serve this with a 1-tablespoon (15 g) side of mashed Oh So Sweet Potato Purée (page 34) or Ready, Set, Go Avocado Purée (page 30).

1 tablespoon (11 g) cooked black beans (homemade or canned)

1 tablespoon (10 g) cooked rice

1 teaspoon plain yogurt

1 tablespoon (7 g) grated Cheddar cheese

MICROWAVE METHOD: Warm the beans and rice in a small covered microwave-safe dish for 10 to 20 seconds. Add breast milk, formula, or cooking liquid (if needed) and mash with a fork. Top the beans and rice with the yogurt and cheese.

YIELD: 1 baby serving, or ¼ cup (about 55 g)

EACH SERVING (if using no optional ingredients) CONTAINS: 40.3 calories; 0.6 g total fat; 0.4 grams saturated fat; 1.9 mg cholesterol; 59.4 mg sodium; 5.3 g carbohydrates; 1.1 g dietary fiber; 3.3 g protein; 40.6 mg calcium; 0.4 mg iron; 55.1 IU vitamin A; and 0.0 mg vitamin C.

Pretty Please Peruvian Bean Purée

Lima beans are sometimes called butter beans because of their buttery texture. If you don't have lima beans on hand, try black beans or navy beans.

½ small leek, bulb only

1 tablespoon (14 g) butter

¼ cup (43 g) canned lima beans with about 1 tablespoon (15 ml) liquid

STOVETOP METHOD: Wash and finely slice the bulb of leak. Melt the butter in a small frying pan over medium heat. Add the leek and sauté 3 to 5 minutes, or until tender. Stir in the lima beans and liquid and heat through. Transfer to a small bowl and mash. (For a smoother consistency, purée in blender 20 seconds.)

YIELD: 1 baby serving, or ¼ cup (55 g)

EACH SERVING CONTAINS: 159.5 calories; 11.2 g total fat; 8.1 grams saturated fat; 30.0 mg cholesterol; 3.5 mg sodium; 11.0 g carbohydrates; 3.7 g dietary fiber; 3.8 g protein; 19.4 mg calcium; 1.4 mg iron; 763.9 IU vitamin A; and 5.7 mg vitamin C.

Scrumptious Scrambled Egg Yolk with Cottage Cheese

Consider serving this recipe with some skinless apple quarters. Lightly dust the fruit with a bit of cinnamon for a new flavor sensation!

1 tablespoon (14 g) whole milk cottage cheese

1 egg yolk

1 teaspoon olive oil

STOVETOP METHOD: Mix the cottage cheese and egg yolk in a small cup and beat well with a fork. Heat the oil in a frying pan over medium heat. Add the egg-cheese mixture and scramble until the egg is well cooked.

YIELD: 1 baby serving, or 3 tablespoons (45 g)

EACH SERVING CONTAINS: 110.9 calories; 9.8 g total fat; 2.7 grams saturated fat; 212.9 mg cholesterol; 63.2 mg sodium; 1.4 g carbohydrates; 0.0 g dietary fiber; 4.2 g protein; 31.9 mg calcium; 0.5 mg iron; 270.1 IU vitamin A; and 0.0 mg vitamin C.

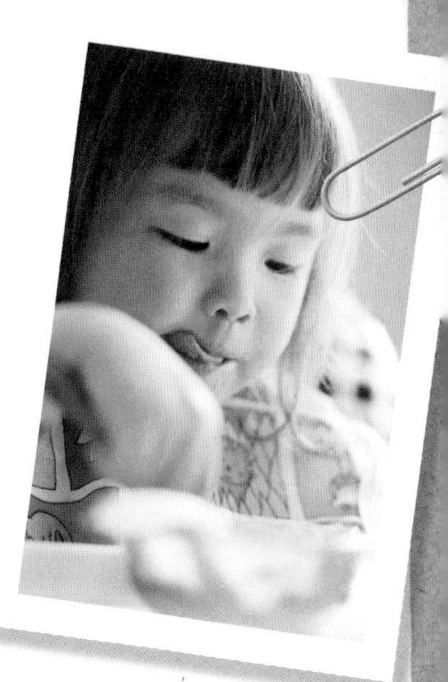

Refried Beans with Cheddar Cheese

The olive oil in this recipe provides added calories for your growing baby. Consider serving with a side of mashed avocado.

2 tablespoons (32 g) canned full-fat refried beans

1 tablespoon (7 g) grated Cheddar cheese

½ teaspoon olive oil

2 teaspoons sour cream

STOVETOP METHOD: In a small frying pan over medium heat, combine the beans, cheese, and oil. Cook until the mixture is warm and the cheese is melted. Top with sour cream.

YIELD: 1 baby serving, or ¼ cup (about 55 g)

EACH SERVING CONTAINS: 81.0 calories; 4.8 g total fat; 1.7 grams saturated fat; 7.9 mg cholesterol; 103.3 mg sodium; 5.1 g carbohydrates; 2.0 g dietary fiber; 3.8 g protein; 43.0 mg calcium; 0.6 mg iron; 116.7 IU vitamin A; and 0.0 mg vitamin C.

Super Silly Fusilli with Zucchini and Carrots

Kids love pasta, and pasta and vegetables go well together. The combinations are endless, and you can experiment with different types and sizes of pasta and a variety of vegetables to discover your baby's favorite.

¼ small zucchini

2 baby carrots

½ cup (70 g) cooked whole wheat fusilli (corkscrew) pasta

¼ cup (25 g) grated Parmesan or Pecorino Romano cheese

MICROWAVE METHOD: Trim and chop zucchini and chop carrots. Cook zucchini and carrots in small amount of water for 2 minutes. Drain and add the vegetables to the cooked pasta along with the cheese. Stir well.

YIELD: 5 baby servings, ¼ cup (55 g) each

EACH SERVING CONTAINS: 37.8 calories; 1.3 g total fat; 0.7 grams saturated fat; 3.5 mg cholesterol; 73.6 mg sodium; 4.5 g carbohydrates; 0.6 g dietary fiber; 2.4 g protein; 57.3 mg calcium; 0.2 mg iron; 1108.8 IU vitamin A; and 0.7 mg vitamin C.

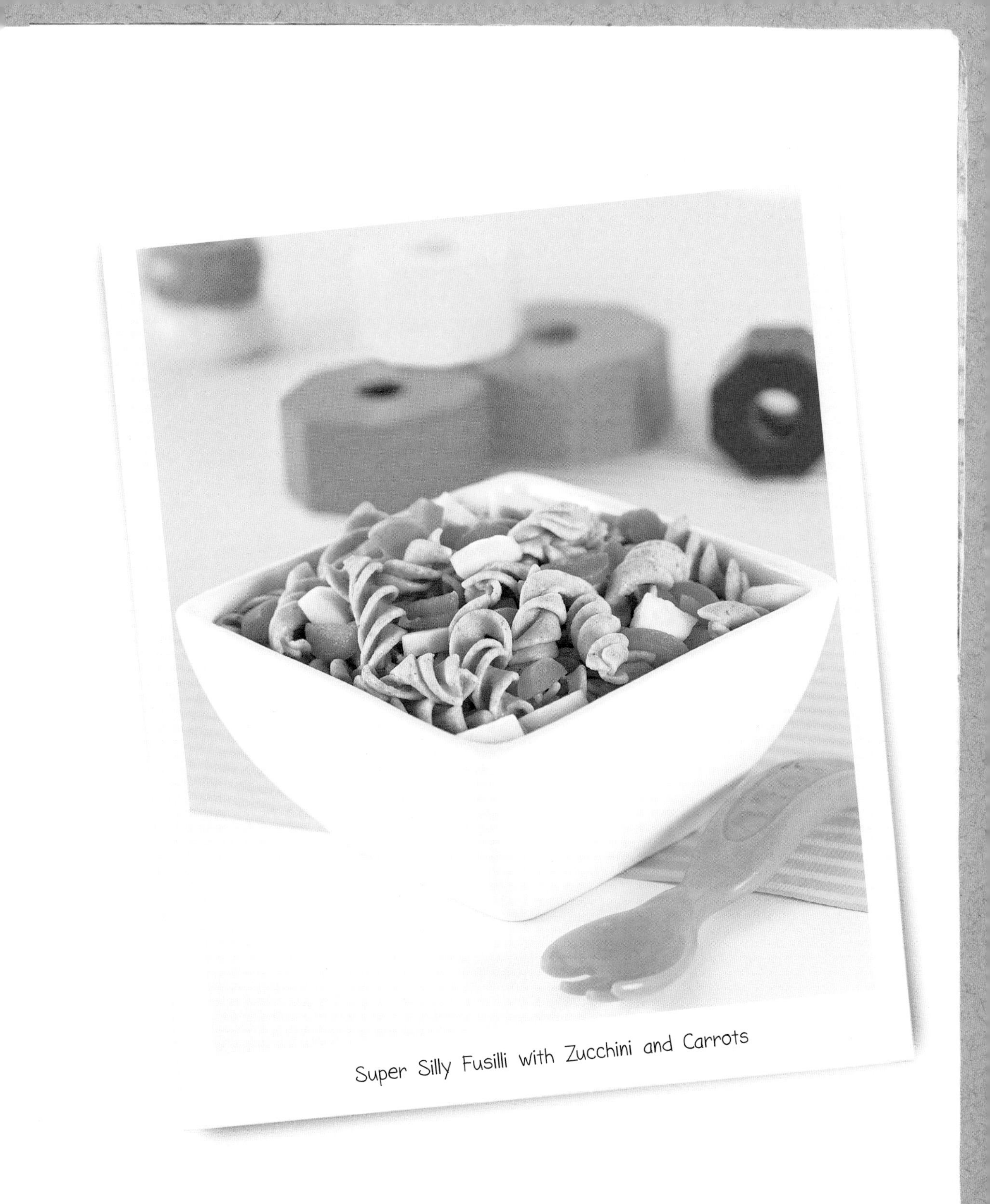

Super Silly Fusilli with Zucchini and Carrots

Baby's First Raisin Purée

This very sweet purée is made with dark, seedless raisins. Commercially grown raisins are sometimes treated with sulfites to extend their shelf life, so buy organic raisins for this reason. Your baby will love their natural sweetness! Storing raisins in an airtight container and keeping them in the refrigerator will extend their freshness and prevent them from drying out.

1/4 cup (35 g) dark, seedless organic raisins

1/4 cup (60 ml) water

MICROWAVE METHOD: Place the raisins and water in a microwave-safe dish. Microwave on high for 40 seconds until hot. Allow to cool slightly and then transfer to a blender and purée 30 to 60 seconds until smooth. (You may need to scrape the raisins down with a spatula.)

YIELD: 1 baby serving, or 1/4 cup (55 g)

EACH SERVING CONTAINS: 130.0 calories; 0.0 g total fat; 0.0 grams saturated fat; 0.0 mg cholesterol; 10.0 mg sodium; 31.0 g carbohydrates; 2.0 g dietary fiber; 1.0 g protein; 20.0 mg calcium; 1.1 mg iron; 0.0 IU vitamin A; and 0.0 mg vitamin C.

All-Occasion Raisin Purée

Raisins are a good source of iron and make a nutritious snack for babies and toddlers. However, dried raisins can cause choking; they also stick to teeth and can cause cavities. Avoid these problems by soaking raisins in hot water until they become plump and soft, then chop or purée them, thinning the purée as neccessary with the water they were soaked in. Puréed raisins can be spread on crackers, bread, waffles, and pancakes, served with yogurt or cream cheese, or added to milk shakes or smoothies. Raisins can also be cooked with foods such as rice, oatmeal cereals, or added to bread pudding for a yummy treat.

Baby's Second Raisin Purée

This purée is made with golden, seedless raisins and is mellow and less sweet that Baby's First Raisin Purée. The iron content is the same in both dark and golden raisins.

1/4 cup (35 g) golden, seedless organic raisins

3 tablespoons (45 ml) hot water

Place the raisins and water in a blender. Purée 1 minute until smooth. (You may need to scrape the raisins down with a spatula.)

YIELD: 1 baby serving, or 1/4 cup (about 55 g)

EACH SERVING CONTAINS: 130.0 calories; 0.0 g total fat; 0.0 grams saturated fat; 0.0 mg cholesterol; 10.0 mg sodium; 31.0 g carbohydrates; 2.0 g dietary fiber; 1.0 g protein; 20.0 mg calcium; 1.1 mg iron; 0.0 IU vitamin A; and 0.0 mg vitamin C.

Carrot, Apple, and Raisin Delight

At this age, most babies have the dexterity and coordination to handle cooked raisins. Just be sure they are soft and plump to avoid the risk of choking.

½ apple

1 tablespoon (15 ml) vegetable oil

1 cup (122 g) sliced carrots

¼ cup (35 g) raisins

½ cup (120 ml) water

STOVETOP METHOD: Peel, core, and finely chop the apple. Heat the oil in a medium saucepan over low heat. Add the carrots and sauté 5 minutes. Add the apple, raisins, and water; cover and simmer 10 minutes or until the carrots are soft.

YIELD: 5 baby servings, ¼ cup (55 g) each

EACH SERVING CONTAINS: 52.2 calories; 1.0 g total fat; 0.2 grams saturated fat; 0.0 mg cholesterol; 19.8 mg sodium; 10.7 g carbohydrates; 1.5 g dietary fiber; 0.5 g protein; 13.3 mg calcium; 0.3 mg iron; 4284.8 IU vitamin A; and 2.2 mg vitamin C.

Yummy-in-My-Tummy Raisin Smoothie

Smoothies can be a wonderful source of concentrated nutrients and calories. If ever your child throws a tantrum and refuses solid food, try blending her favorite fruits and veggies together for a "save the day" meal she can drink!

2 tablespoons (28 g) Baby's First Raisin Purée (page 112)

½ banana

1 cup (235 ml) breast milk or formula

Place the Baby's First Raisin Purée, banana, and breast milk or formula in a blender and process until smooth.

YIELD: 4 baby servings, ¼ cup (55 g) each

EACH SERVING (if using breast milk) CONTAINS: 65.5 calories; 2.8 g total fat; 1.3 grams saturated fat; 8.6 mg cholesterol; 11.3 mg sodium; 9.8 g carbohydrates; 0.5 g dietary fiber; 0.9 g protein; 21.9 mg calcium; 0.1 mg iron; 140.0 IU vitamin A; and 4.4 mg vitamin C.

Love Those Smoothies!

There's a nice selection of smoothies, shakes, and yogurt drinks in this cookbook. That's because babies and toddlers sometimes have small and capricious appetites, and a lot of nutrition from several food groups can be packed into a small, healthy drink that your child may accept. During teething, these cool drinks are often preferable to solids.

Super Simple Cooked Beets

This is a simple way to cook beets to use in a wide variety of recipes.

4 small beets

MICROWAVE METHOD: Trim and scrub beets. Place them in a microwave-safe bowl with a small amount of water. Cover and microwave on high 15 to 20 minutes or until the beets are soft. Cool and slip off the peel.

YIELD: 2 baby servings, 2 beets each

EACH SERVING CONTAINS: 44.0 calories; 0.2 g total fat; 0.0 grams saturated fat; 0.0 mg cholesterol; 77.0 mg sodium; 10.0 g carbohydrates; 2.0 g dietary fiber; 1.7 g protein; 16.0 mg calcium; 0.8 mg iron; 35.0 IU vitamin A; and 3.6 mg vitamin C.

You Can't Beat Beets!

Beets, a good source of folic acid, are naturally sweet and pleasing to babies. Baking or roasting beets brings out their sweetness and flavor. Note that dark purple beets can be messy, so don't be alarmed if your baby's diapers turn red! There are other varieties available, including yellow and white, and they taste even sweeter than the red ones. All are recommended. Your baby may enjoy beets plain or lightly mashed with butter. Plain yogurt or sour cream is also delicious with beets. Beet greens are the most nutritious part of the beet plant, and they are high in potassium, beta-carotene, and folic acid. The tops can be cooked and prepared like other greens, sautéed, steamed, or microwaved with a bit of water.

Beet, Avocado, and Pear Rainbow

The colors in this dish make it appealing to babies. The pear can be optional if your baby prefers a more savory recipe.

1/4 cup (55 g) peeled and mashed cooked beets (page 114)

1/4 cup (55 g) mashed avocado

1/4 ripe pear

Place the mashed beet on one side of a baby bowl and the mashed avocado on the other. Top with thin slices of peeled and cored ripe pear.

YIELD: 2 baby servings, 1/4 cup (55 g) each

EACH SERVING CONTAINS: 56.4 calories; 3.0 g total fat; 0.6 grams saturated fat; 0.0 mg cholesterol; 58.3 mg sodium; 7.5 g carbohydrates; 2.6 g dietary fiber; 1.0 g protein; 5.0 mg calcium; 0.3 mg iron; 47.1 IU vitamin A; and 6.2 mg vitamin C.

Perfect Polenta with Cheddar

This is a mild and sweet dish that babies will love. Made in the microwave, it has a soft consistency. Soon, when your baby is a year old, you may be changing from breast milk or formula to whole milk.

1/2 cup (120 ml) breast milk or formula

1 tablespoon (9 g) white cornmeal

1 tablespoon (7 g) mild Cheddar cheese

MICROWAVE METHOD: Place the breast milk or formula and cornmeal in a microwave-safe bowl. Microwave on high 2 minutes. Stir and microwave 2 minutes longer or until the cornmeal has a soft pudding consistency. Stir with a fork and whip in the cheese. Let cool slightly before serving.

YIELD: 3 baby servings, 1/4 cup each

EACH SERVING (if using breast milk) CONTAINS: 40.8 calories; 1.5 g total fat; 0.8 grams saturated fat; 4.5 mg cholesterol; 34.6 mg sodium; 4.6 g carbohydrates; 0.2 g dietary fiber; 2.2 g protein; 54.3 mg calcium; 0.1 mg iron; 58.2 IU vitamin A; and 0.0 mg vitamin C.

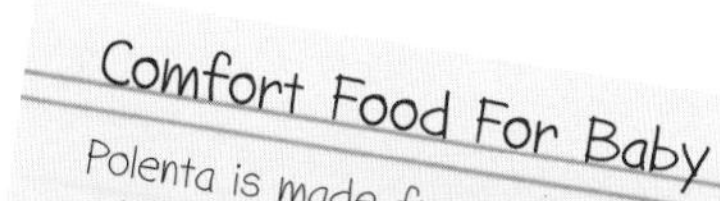

Comfort Food For Baby

Polenta is made from cornmeal, has a soft texture, a bland flavor, and is a soothing meal for babies. Served with flavorful sauces, vegetables, or cheese, it's also a satisfying and delicious food for adults. Ready-made polenta is now available in most grocery stores. Packed in water in a tube, it comes ready to slice, heat, and serve. Microwaving keeps it very moist. When sautéed in a skillet, it becomes crisp on the outside.

Elbow Macaroni with Peas and Parmesan

This is a finger food favorite for babies. Whole wheat pasta can also be used.

1 to 2 tablespoons (14 to 28 g) butter

¼ cup (25 g) grated Parmesan or Pecorino Romano cheese

½ cup (70 g) cooked elbow macaroni

½ cup (75 g) fresh or (65 g) frozen peas

STOVETOP METHOD: Add the butter and cheese to warm macaroni and peas and stir until the butter is melted and the cheese is well mixed.

YIELD: 5 baby servings, ¼ cup (55 g) each

EACH SERVING CONTAINS: 59.1 calories; 3.5 g total fat; 2.3 grams saturated fat; 9.5 mg cholesterol; 68.9 mg sodium; 4.1 g carbohydrates; 0.7 g dietary fiber; 2.6 g protein; 53.4 mg calcium; 0.3 mg iron; 175.0 IU vitamin A; and 0.9 mg vitamin C.

Itsy-Bitsy Apricot Chicken with Couscous

Couscous is a coarsely ground semolina pasta. It's like a blank canvas that takes on the flavors of the foods you cook it with.

1 small, skinless, boneless chicken breast or chicken tender

¼ cup (39 g) cooked couscous

1 tablespoon (15 g) Naturally Sweet Apricot Purée (page 56)

MICROWAVE METHOD: Cook and dice chicken. In a small, microwave-safe bowl, combine all ingredients. Microwave until warm and serve.

YIELD: 2 baby servings, ¼ cup (55 g) each

EACH SERVING CONTAINS: 109.4 calories; 5.1 g total fat; 1.1 grams saturated fat; 12.5 mg cholesterol; 130.7 mg sodium; 10.3 g carbohydrates; 0.7 g dietary fiber; 5.3 g protein; 7.4 mg calcium; 0.5 mg iron; 90.9 IU vitamin A; and 0.0 mg vitamin C.

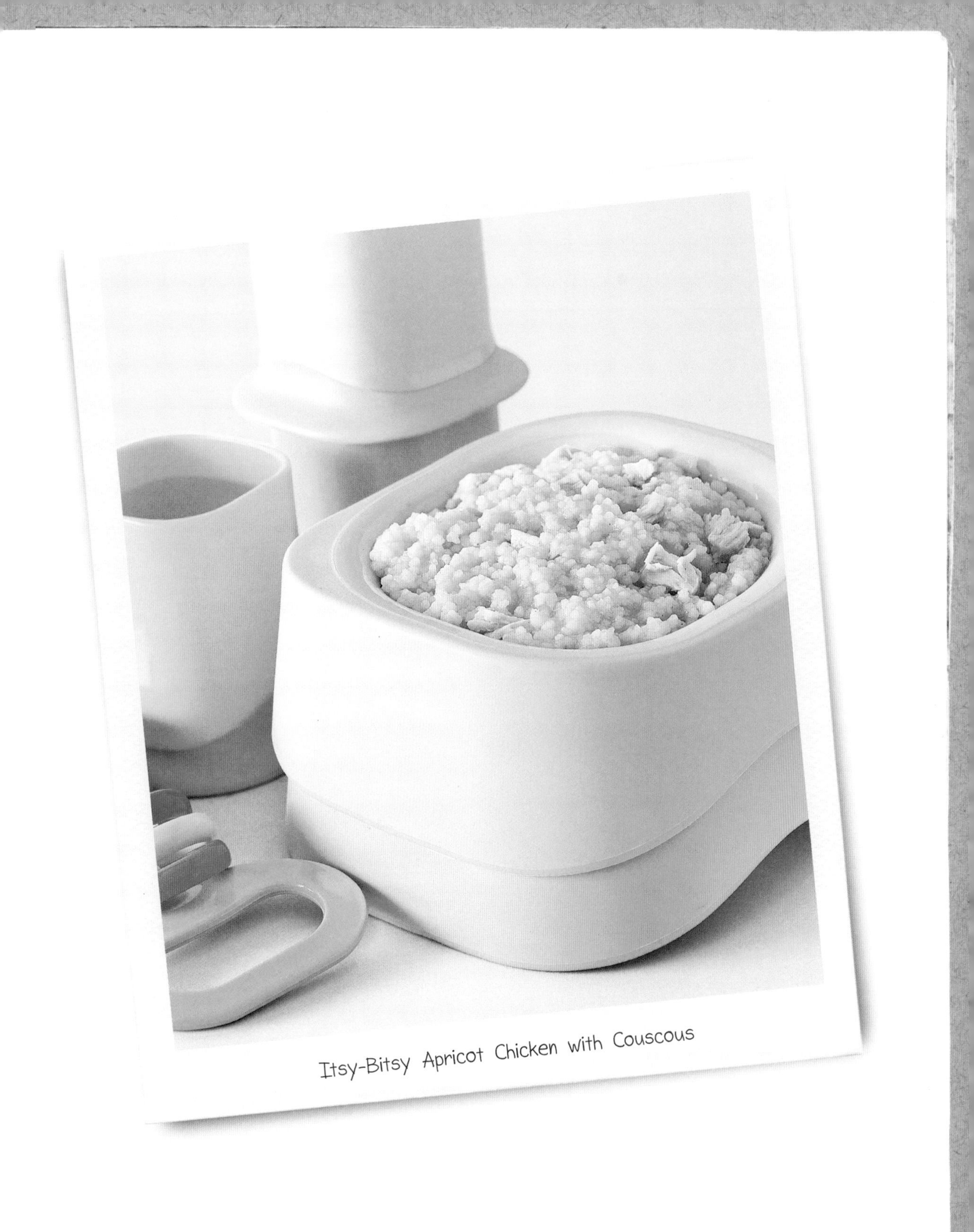

Itsy-Bitsy Apricot Chicken with Couscous

Tasty Tofu and Egg Yolk Treat

This meal is packed with protein and tastes divine!

1 teaspoon unsalted butter

2 tablespoons (1 ounce, or 28 g) silken tofu

1 egg yolk

1 teaspoon milk

1 teaspoon grated Parmesan cheese

STOVETOP METHOD: Heat the butter in a small frying pan over medium heat. Mash the tofu. In a small bowl, whisk the tofu and egg yolk together. Add the milk and cheese and whisk until well blended. Pour into the frying pan and scramble until well done.

YIELD: 1 baby serving, or 1/4 cup (55 g)

EACH SERVING CONTAINS: 115.8 calories; 9.8 g total fat; 4.9 grams saturated fat; 223.6 mg cholesterol; 45.2 mg sodium; 1.2 g carbohydrates; 0.0 g dietary fiber; 4.8 g protein; 79.5 mg calcium; 0.7 mg iron; 417.0 IU vitamin A; and 0.0 mg vitamin C.

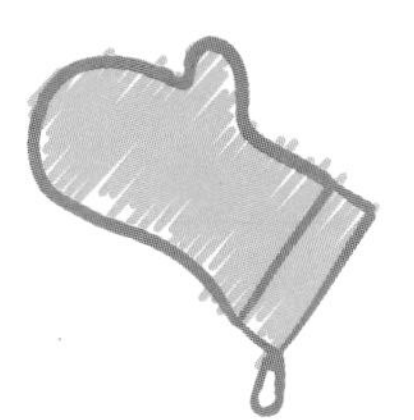

Cream Cheese-Pineapple Finger Sandwich Fun

Add variety to this finger sandwich by changing the bread. English muffins and Challah bread are great choices.

1 tablespoon (15 g) cream cheese

1 tablespoon (15 g) puréed fresh pineapple

1/2 slice oatmeal bread

Whip the cream cheese with a fork. Mix in the pineapple purée and spread on the bread. Fold the bread over and cut into small pieces.

YIELD: 1 baby serving, or 1 finger sandwich

EACH SERVING CONTAINS: 93.4 calories; 5.7 g total fat; 2.9 grams saturated fat; 16.0 mg cholesterol; 127.9 mg sodium; 8.8 g carbohydrates; 1.2 g dietary fiber; 2.2 g protein; 25.7 mg calcium; 0.4 mg iron; 185.6 IU vitamin A; and 3.1 mg vitamin C.

Pineapple-Banana-Blueberry Delight

This is a healthy and refreshing dessert. If your baby is teething, lightly freeze the fruit before serving and offer as finger food. It will soothe sore gums.

5 small (1 x 1-inch, or 2.5 x 2.5 cm) chunks of pineapple

2 tablespoons (28 g) lightly mashed banana

2 tablespoons (18 g) lightly crushed blueberries

Cut pineapple into very small pieces and lightly mash. Place the mashed pineapple, banana, and blueberries in a bowl and feed with a small spoon.

YIELD: 3 baby servings, 1⁄4 cup (55 g) each

EACH SERVING CONTAINS: 25.0 calories; 0.1 g total fat; 0.0 grams saturated fat; 0.0 mg cholesterol; 0.6 mg sodium; 6.4 g carbohydrates; 0.7 g dietary fiber; 0.3 g protein; 7.0 mg calcium; 0.2 mg iron; 24.9 IU vitamin A; and 4.6 mg vitamin C.

Raspberry Kiwi Melon Cup

Raspberries are fragrantly sweet yet tart at the same time. They are also high in good-for-you flavinoids.

1 thick (2 x 2 inch, or 5 x 5 cm) slice cantaloupe

5 raspberries

5 small pieces kiwi fruit

With a spoon, scoop out enough of the cantaloupe slice to make a cup for the berries and kiwi fruit. Chop the scooped-out cantaloupe into small pieces and mix with the raspberries and kiwi. Spoon the fruits into the cantaloupe cup.

YIELD: 2 baby servings, 1⁄4 cup (55 g) each

EACH SERVING CONTAINS: 26.2 calories; 0.2 g total fat; 0.3 grams saturated fat; 0.0 mg cholesterol; 8.4 mg sodium; 6.6 g carbohydrates; 0.7 g dietary fiber; 0.6 g protein; 9.1 mg calcium; 0.2 mg iron; 1733.1 IU vitamin A; and 29.0 mg vitamin C.

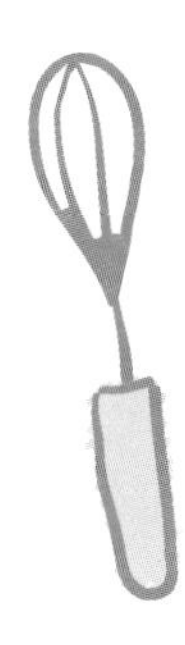

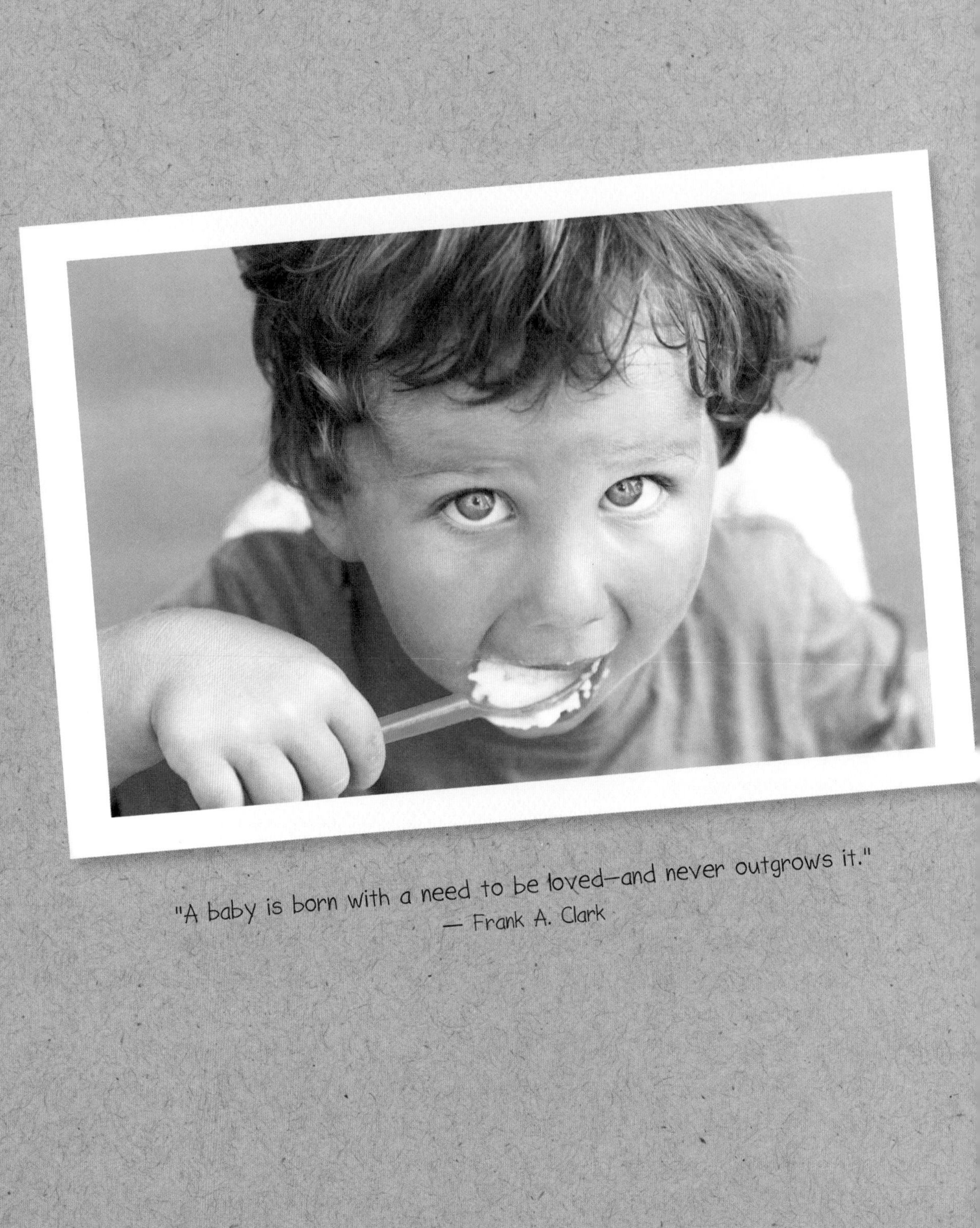

"A baby is born with a need to be loved—and never outgrows it."
— Frank A. Clark

CHAPTER THREE

Feeding Your Toddler the Best—from Twelve to Twenty-Three Months

Now that your baby is one year old, he can start sharing family meals. So, the recipe format you've been following will change at bit. In this chapter you'll find recipes categorized by day-part (breakfast, lunch, and dinner) in addition to healthy snack ideas that your toddler might enjoy. Keep in mind, all the toddler recipes can be given anytime between twelve and twenty-three months—and sometimes beyond—and you can continue to use your little one's favorite baby recipes; just offer larger servings and chunkier textures.

During the toddler years, you'll see your baby's self-feeding improve, and she should be able to take all liquids from a cup (with help at first, of course). Don't be overly concerned if there is a sharp drop in appetite around your baby's first birthday. This is quite common and could last until about eighteen months of age.

Secrets to Success at Mealtime: Helpful Hints You Need to Know

Up to this point, your baby has been eating wholesome, nutritious foods and enjoying them, so you've successfully established a healthy eating platform. To build on this foundation, continue to select fresh foods and try to resist processed and fast foods. The recipes in this section are also quick and easy to make, not to mention fun and delicious for your toddler to eat, so forge ahead! You're doing a great job!

BE CONSISTENT WITH MEALS AND SNACKS

Since a toddler's stomach is about the size of your fist, serve three small meals—breakfast, lunch, and dinner—and two or three small snacks during the day. Consistency with meals and snacks is important since it provides a foundation for good eating habits and is just as important as sleep time or nap time.

If your toddler becomes fussy about what he's fed, try preparing the same food different ways. For example, if your child refuses mashed sweet potato for lunch, try serving Better-for-Baby Sweet Potato Fries (page 60) the next day as a snack. If he does not want to eat beans, try hummus spread on crackers. Most important, don't bribe your baby with games or dessert. That won't help the situation and might actually create eating issues later. Just be patient, and give your child time to eat his meals.

KEEP AN EYE ON ALLERGIES

When your baby turns one year old, the danger of food intolerance or allergy decreases, but continue to watch for rashes or diarrhea after introducing a new food. (See "Understanding Allergies and Food Intolerance," page 209). If there is no history of allergies in your family, you can start to give your toddler the following:

- Citrus fruits
- Honey nut butters
- Mangoes
- Spices and herbs—but use them sparingly and in small amounts since many things are still brand new to your toddler
- Strawberries
- Tomatoes
- Whole eggs

DO NOT RESTRICT FAT AND CHOLESTEROL

Babies need fat in their diets for brain growth and development, and they get all they need from breast milk or formula. But as babies grow into toddlers, their nutrition requirements change. They have tiny stomachs and need foods that are calorie dense. Since snacks and meal portions are small, whole milk, whole-fat dairy products, and other fatty foods are necessary to provide essential calories. In fact, half of a toddler's calories should come from fat, so do not limit fatty foods, including full-fat cow's milk, which usually can be given instead of breast milk or formula after one year of age.

According to the American Heart Association, fat and cholesterol should not be restricted in the diets of children under age two. Babies and toddlers require more fat in their diets than older children and adults, and cholesterol is essential for babies' growth. Children from one to two years old should be given whole milk and whole-milk products, which contain the necessary amount of cholesterol for this age group. (In fact, breast milk has more cholesterol than whole cow's milk.)

It's important to note that high levels of saturated fat in an adult's diet can cause elevated cholesterol, which may increase the risk of cardiovascular disease, heart attack, and stroke. Because of this, health experts regularly encourage adults to limit their intake of dietary cholesterol and saturated fat.

The family's best insurance against consuming too much cholesterol and saturated fat is to eat a balanced diet rich in grains, vegetables, and fruit. Some lean meat, poultry, or fish, alternating or combined with legumes and low or nonfat dairy products, will give adults and children over two all the fat and cholesterol they need.

OFFER WHOLE MILK WITH MEALS

Some mothers may choose to continue breast-feeding. For those who don't, begin serving ¼ to ½ cup (60 to 120 ml) of whole milk with meals. You can decide how much milk to serve with each meal or snack, as long as your toddler gets at least 2 cups (475 ml) of whole milk every day.

EXPAND YOUR TODDLER'S CEREAL CHOICES

Your toddler should continue to eat cooked cereals. Instead of ground baby cereal, you can now serve traditional cream of wheat, oatmeal, rice, barley, and grits.

KEEP THE VEGGIES COMING

Hopefully, your toddler will continue to enjoy all the vegetables she was given as a baby. For the toddler who refuses to eat vegetables, some parents mix cooked, puréed carrots into tomato sauce and steamed puréed spinach into pesto sauce. You might find that this works well for the child who loves pasta but not carrots and spinach. If you have a juicer, make carrot juice and mix it with other juice or make carrot purée and use it in smoothies. And don't be afraid to offer your toddler foods seasoned with fresh herbs. Basil and parsley are full of vitamins and minerals.

MAKE FRUIT YOUR CHILD'S ONLY "DESSERT"

This book doesn't include recipes for cakes and cookies. The desserts recommended include fresh fruit, sherbet, and fruit sorbets. Although these particular desserts are considered "sweets," they do contribute to good nutrition and healthy eating habits. If your baby enjoys fruit, it may well become a lifelong preference over candy, chocolate, cakes, or cookies. Buy the best quality fruit you can find, because the flavor and sweetness will appeal to your child.

What's Important about Baby's One-Year Checkup?

When your baby becomes a toddler at age one, she will probably have more or less tripled her birth weight, stand about 29 inches (74 cm) tall, and have six or eight teeth. An annual assessment of a child's weight and height gives important indicators of normal growth, as does measuring the head circumference. The most rapid and critical period of human brain growth begins at conception and continues into the second year. Brain cells increase in number until the child is twelve to fifteen months old and increase thereafter in mass and size. Although growth slows, babies become stronger and more coordinated.

PREFECTLY BALANCED BOWLS AND PLATES:

RECIPES FOR TWELVE TO SEVENTEEN MONTHS

Healthy doesn't have to mean repetitive or boring, so you might be surprised to see all the varied and delicious recipes in this section. In many cases, breakfast recipes can make wonderful lunches, and lunch recipes can be enjoyed for a snack. As your child becomes more independent, remain flexible. Think about mini-sandwiches for a quick breakfast or an egg scramble for a protein-packed dinner. By using a little creativity, your toddler will never tire of healthy food.

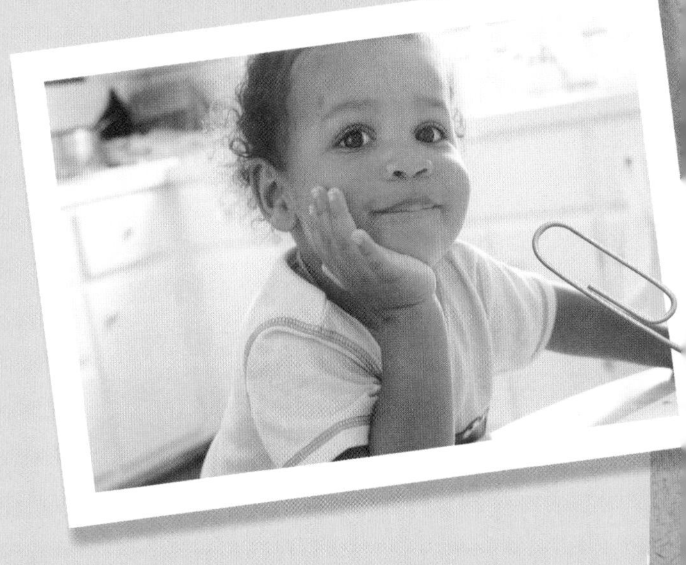

Yummy Yogurt Cone Sundae

Feel free to substitute other fresh fruit that your baby might enjoy. Thin slices of strawberries and kiwi are a delightful combination!

1⁄3 banana

1⁄4 cup (36 g) fresh blueberries

1⁄4 cup (60 g) plain yogurt

1 ice cream waffle bowl

Lightly mash the banana and blueberries. Place the yogurt in the ice-cream waffle bowl and top with the banana and blueberries.

YIELD: 1 toddler serving, or 1 sundae

EACH SERVING CONTAINS: 143.5 calories; 3.2 g total fat; 1.3 grams saturated fat; 8.0 mg cholesterol; 54.0 mg sodium; 27.2 g carbohydrates; 1.9 g dietary fiber; 3.8 g protein; 78.3 mg calcium; 1.0 mg iron; 105.8 IU vitamin A; and 7.3 mg vitamin C.

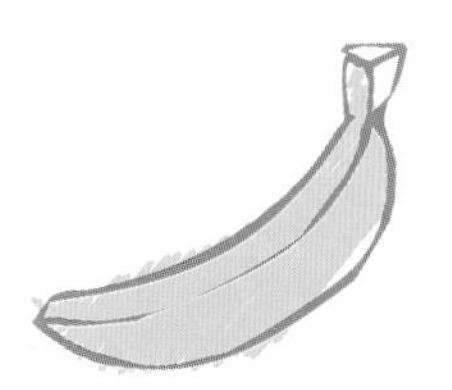

Super Scrambled Egg and Turkey

Consider serving this yummy breakfast with 1⁄2 cup (120 ml) of milk.

1⁄2 teaspoon olive oil

1 egg

1⁄2 precooked turkey or vegetable sausage link

STOVETOP METHOD: Heat the oil in a small skillet over low heat. Lightly beat the egg; pour into the pan. Stir occasionally until the egg is well cooked. Put egg on a plate and set aside. In the same skillet, add the sausage link and cook 1 1⁄2 minutes until warmed through. (Check to make sure it is not too hot before serving.)

YIELD: 1 toddler serving

EACH SERVING (if using turkey sausage) CONTAINS: 151.0 calories; 10.8 g total fat; 3.1 grams saturated fat; 242.5 mg cholesterol; 280 mg sodium; 1.5 g carbohydrates; 0.0 g dietary fiber; 12.0 g protein; 20.0 mg calcium; 0.7 mg iron; 300.0 IU vitamin A; and 0.0 mg vitamin C.

Stupendous Strawberry Tofu and Prune Smoothie

You can find all-natural strawberry silken tofu in the refrigerated section of your grocery store. Plain silken tofu can also work in this recipe.

8 pitted, ready-to-eat prunes (sometimes called dried plums)

¼ cup (60 g) strawberry silken tofu

Put ingredients into blender and liquefy.

YIELD: 1 toddler serving

EACH SERVING CONTAINS: 172.5 calories; 1.5 g total fat; 0.0 grams saturated fat; 0.0 mg cholesterol; 4.1 mg sodium; 38.9 g carbohydrates; 5.2 g dietary fiber; 3.7 g protein; 60.8 mg calcium; 1.0 mg iron; 1096.7 IU vitamin A; and 3.9 mg vitamin C.

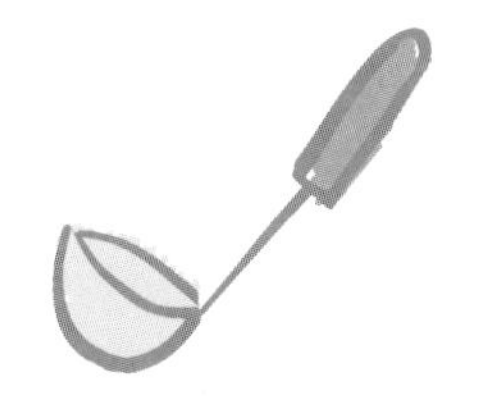

Baby's First Rice Pudding

This will be baby's first taste of real rice pudding. It will also be good for little ones attempting to feed themselves as the pudding clings nicely to the spoon. Take out baby's serving and share the rest with the family for a treat!

3 cups (705 ml) milk

½ cup (93 g) uncooked long grain rice

¼ cup (50 g) granulated sugar

1 cinnamon stick

¼ teaspoon vanilla extract

¼ cup (35 g) chopped raisins

STOVETOP METHOD: In a small stockpot over medium-high heat, combine milk, rice, sugar, and cinnamon stick and bring to a boil. Lower heat and cook, uncovered, stirring occasionally, for 25 minutes or until rice is creamy and tender. Stir in the vanilla. Remove from heat, add raisins, and discard cinnamon stick. Cover and let stand for 10 minutes. Serve warm.

YIELD: 9 baby servings, ¼ cup (55 g) each

EACH SERVING CONTAINS: 123.0 calories; 2.6 g total fat; 1.5 grams saturated fat; 8.1 mg cholesterol; 33.7 mg sodium; 21.2 g carbohydrates; 0.2 g dietary fiber; 3.6 g protein; 100.0 mg calcium; 0.5mg iron; 83.0 IU vitamin A; and 0.0 mg vitamin C.

Strawberry-Banana-Tofu Smoothie

Tofu contains all eight essential amino acids and is a rich source of protein. If you don't have strawberries on hand for this recipe, peaches work well also.

1 small banana

6 large fresh or frozen strawberries

1/3 cup (1/4 package, or 80 g) silken tofu

1 cup (235 ml) whole milk

Lightly mash the banana. Hull and quarter the strawberries. Combine all ingredients in blender and process until smooth.

YIELD: 4 toddler servings, 1/2 cup (120 ml) each

EACH SERVING CONTAINS: 80.7 calories; 2.6 g total fat; 1.2 grams saturated fat; 6.1 mg cholesterol; 25.0 mg sodium; 11.8 g carbohydrates; 1.3 g dietary fiber; 3.3 g protein; 87.1 mg calcium; 0.4 mg iron; 84.3 IU vitamin A; and 18.4 mg vitamin C.

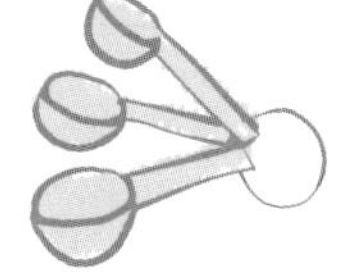

Baby's First Blueberry Bread Pudding

Introducing your little one to different flavors is just as important as introducing him to various textures. By doing this, he'll become a more adventurous and less fussy eater.

1 cup (225 g) crumbled blueberry muffins

1 egg

1/2 cup (120 ml) whole milk

2 teaspoons butter

1 tablespoon (15 g) brown sugar

1/3 cup (52 g) frozen blueberries

OVEN METHOD: Preheat the oven to 350°F (180°C, gas mark 4). Butter a 2-cup (475 ml) ovenproof ramekin. Place the crumbled muffin in the prepared ramekin. In a small bowl, beat the egg and milk together and pour over the muffin. Dot with butter and sprinkle with brown sugar. Top with blueberries. Bake 40 minutes. Cool slightly before serving.

YIELD: 4 toddler servings, 1/2 cup (115 g) each

EACH SERVING CONTAINS: 118.8 calories; 5.0 g total fat; 2.3 grams saturated fat; 61.8 mg cholesterol; 99.5 mg sodium; 15.3 g carbohydrates; 1.1 g dietary fiber; 3.7 g protein; 41.4 mg calcium; 0.5 mg iron; 172.8 IU vitamin A; and 0.2 mg vitamin C.

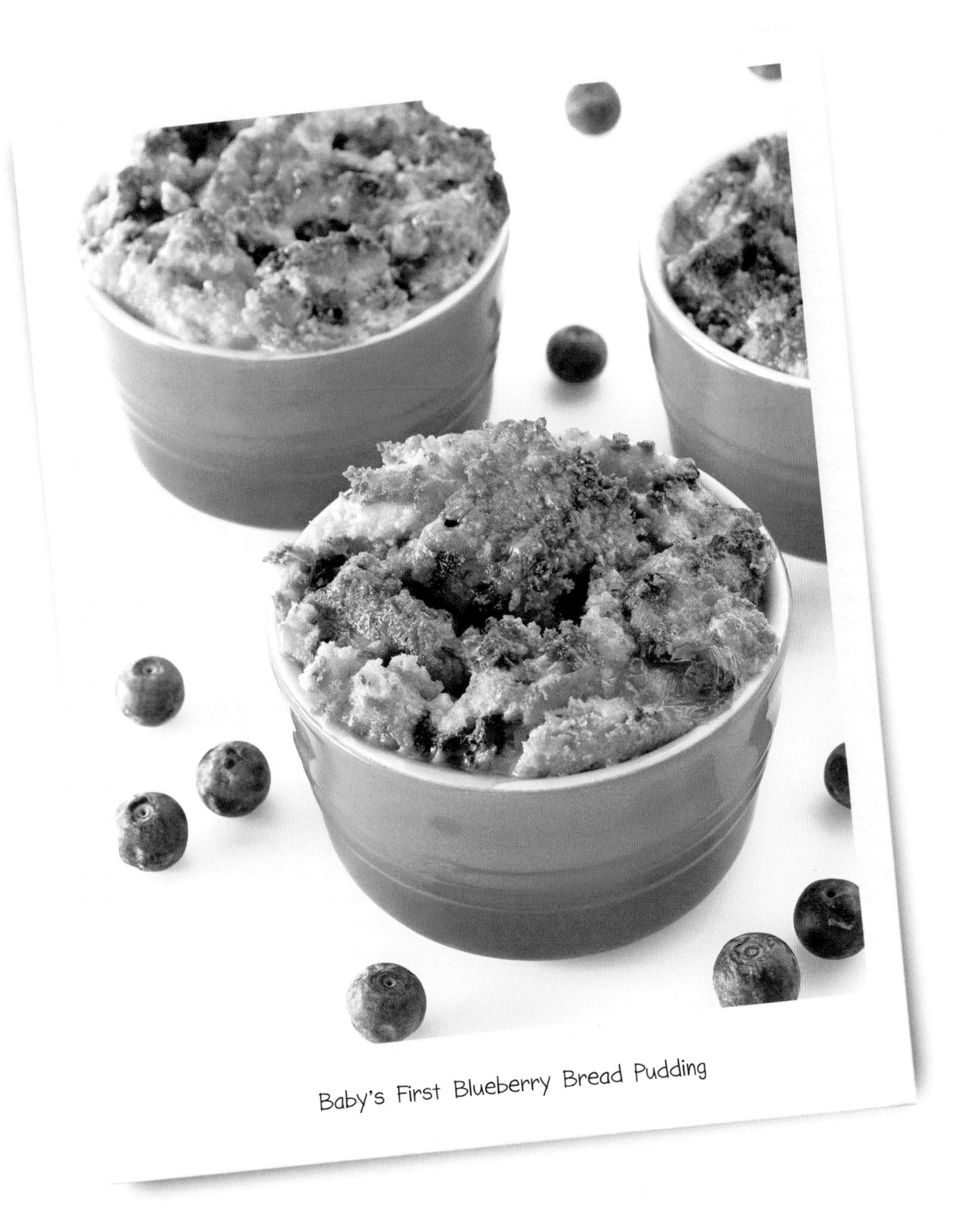

Baby's First Blueberry Bread Pudding

Crunchy Fruit and Cereal Parfait

This recipe offers a satisfying mix of flavors and textures for your toddler.

2 tablespoons (16 g) fresh raspberries

2 tablespoons (30 g) plain or vanilla whole-milk yogurt

2 tablespoons (28 g) nut-like cereal nuggets

In a plastic baby cup, layer 1 tablespoon (8 g) raspberries, 1 tablespoon (15 g) yogurt, 1 tablespoon (14 g) cereal; repeat with remaining ingredients. Let the parfait sit for a few minutes before serving, so the cereal can soften.

YIELD: 2 toddler servings, 3 tablespoons each (about 45 g)

EACH SERVING (if using plain yogurt) CONTAINS: 21.2 calories; 0.6 g total fat; 0.3 grams saturated fat; 2.0 mg cholesterol; 18.7 mg sodium; 3.7 g carbohydrates; 0.2 g dietary fiber; 0.8 g protein; 20.7 mg calcium; 0.7 mg iron; 77.7 IU vitamin A; and 1.5 mg vitamin C.

Goldilocks' Porridge

Consider serving this recipe with 1/2 cup (120 ml) warm whole milk dusted with a bit of cinnamon. This also makes a satisfying lunch on a rainy day.

3/4 cup (175 ml) water

3 tablespoons (28 g) quick-cooking hominy grits

1/4 cup (64 g) frozen sweetened sliced strawberries, thawed

STOVETOP METHOD: Bring the water to a boil in a small saucepan. Slowly stir in the grits and strawberries. Cover the pan and reduce the heat to low. Cook 5 to 6 minutes, stirring occasionally. Serve topped with a dot of butter and a little milk, if desired.

YIELD: 1 toddler serving, or 1/2 cup (about 115 g)

EACH SERVING CONTAINS: 148.2 calories; 0.5 g total fat; 0.0 grams saturated fat; 0.0 mg cholesterol; 0.7 mg sodium; 35.4 g carbohydrates; 2.7 g dietary fiber; 2.6 g protein; 7.2 mg calcium; 1.4 mg iron; 17.6 IU vitamin A; and 25.7 mg vitamin C.

Feeding and Eating: A Natural Rhythm

Children are normally rhythmic in their habits, so satisfying their hunger should be in tune with that rhythm. Meals should be served at the same time each day whenever possible. Although this may conflict with adult schedules initially, babies eventually adapt to the rest of the family's mealtimes, probably because they enjoy the social interaction. So don't be concerned if changes occur intermittently in your child's eating pattern. That's normal. Also, fatigue can often be a major factor in loss of appetite. An exhausted child's appetite is seldom restored until he has had a nap or a good night's sleep.

Mmm Mmm Muesli with Yogurt

Muesli is a cold granola-like cereal, originally from Switzerland, that is rich in essential vitamins, minerals, and enzymes. For your toddler, buy muesli without nuts or dry fruit and add fresh fruit or berries instead.

1/4 cup (20 g) muesli cereal

1/4 banana

1 tablespoon (15 g) plain yogurt

1/2 teaspoon honey

Place the cereal in a small bowl. Slice the banana and place on top of the cereal. In a bowl, combine the honey and yogurt and spoon it on top of the cereal.

YIELD: 1 toddler serving, or 1/4 cup (about 55 g)

EACH SERVING CONTAINS: 156.2 calories; 3.6 g total fat; 0.4 grams saturated fat; 2.0 mg cholesterol; 7.4 mg sodium; 31.3 g carbohydrates; 4.8 g dietary fiber; 4.2 g protein; 40.2 mg calcium; 1.2 mg iron; 34.0 IU vitamin A; and 2.7 mg vitamin C.

Strawberry-Blueberry-Tofu Smoothie

This is a fresh and delicious way to get your toddler in the habit of enjoying breakfast! The smoothie is also a smart snack.

1/4 cup (60 g) silken strawberry tofu

1/4 cup (36 g) blueberries

1 cup (235 ml) whole milk

In a blender, combine the tofu, blueberries, and milk. Process until smooth.

YIELD: 4 toddler servings, 1/2 cup (120 ml) each

EACH SERVING CONTAINS: 49.0 calories; 2.3 g total fat; 1.1 grams saturated fat; 6.1 mg cholesterol; 24.5 mg sodium; 4.3 g carbohydrates; 0.2 g dietary fiber; 2.7 g protein; 78.8 mg calcium; 0.2 mg iron; 67.2 IU vitamin A; and 0.9 mg vitamin C.

Tiny But Mighty: Know What Your Toddler Needs

Did you know that toddlers burn about 40 calories a day for every inch in height? That's 1160 calories a day for a 29-inch-tall 18-month-old. That's one of the reasons calorie-dense foods are so important in their diet.

Winnie the Pooh's Favorite Breakfast

Rumor has it that Tigger likes this breakfast too, and it's no wonder. The fruit and honey combination is delicious and nutritious!

1 teaspoon Honey Butter (see right)

1/4 toasted whole-wheat English muffin

1 small piece honeydew melon, chopped into small pieces or lightly mashed

Spread the Honey Butter on the muffin and serve with the melon.

YIELD: 1 toddler serving

EACH SERVING CONTAINS: 116.2 calories; 4.1 g total fat; 2.7 grams saturated fat; 10.0 mg cholesterol; 65.1 mg sodium; 19.0 g carbohydrates; 1.3 g dietary fiber; 1.9 g protein; 7.6 mg calcium; 0.7 mg iron; 195.8 IU vitamin A; and 22.5 mg vitamin C.

Honey Butter

This recipe will keep in the refrigerator three to four days, or you can freeze it for up to one month. You can also use agave nectar in place of the honey.

4 tablespoons (1/2 stick, or 55 g) unsalted butter, room temperature

1 tablespoon (20 g) honey

With an electric mixer, whip the butter until light and creamy. Add the honey and whip until fluffy.

YIELD: Twelve 1-teaspoon servings

EACH SERVING CONTAINS: 38.6 calories; 3.7 g total fat; 2.7 grams saturated fat; 10.0 mg cholesterol; 0.1 mg sodium; 1.4 g carbohydrates; 0.0 g dietary fiber; 0.0 g protein; 0.1 mg calcium; 0.0 mg iron; 133.3 IU vitamin A; and 0.0 mg vitamin C.

Baby's Best Banana Buttermilk Pancakes

These pancakes are delicious for children and adults alike. Consider serving with maple syrup or your toddler's favorite jam and 1⁄4 cup (60 ml) grape juice.

1 cup (235 ml) buttermilk

1 egg

3 tablespoons (45 ml) vegetable oil, plus more for cooking the pancakes

1⁄2 banana

1⁄2 cup (60 g) whole-wheat flour

1⁄4 cup (31 g) all-purpose flour

1⁄4 cup (35 g) cornmeal

1 teaspoon baking soda

1⁄2 teaspoon baking powder

STOVETOP METHOD: Mix the buttermilk, egg, and oil in a large bowl. Cut the banana into small pieces or mash it. Combine the whole-wheat flour, all-purpose flour, cornmeal, baking soda, baking powder, and banana in a smaller bowl. Mix well with a fork. Add the dry ingredients to the wet ingredients and stir just enough to moisten all the ingredients. (Small lumps are okay.)

Heat a griddle or skillet to medium hot or until a drop of water bounces off the surface. Coat lightly with oil. With a 1⁄4-cup (60 ml) measure, pour batter onto hot griddle, making a few pancakes at a time. (If the batter seems too thick, thin by stirring in water, a little at a time.) Spread the batter a bit with the bottom of a spoon. Cook until a few bubbles show on the surface of the pancakes and then turn with a wide spatula and cook until both sides are golden brown. Transfer pancakes to warmed platter. Repeat with remaining batter, coating the griddle with oil each time.

YIELD: 6 toddler servings, one 4-inch (10 cm) pancake each

EACH SERVING CONTAINS: 180.1 calories; 8.8 g total fat; 16.3 grams saturated fat; 39.1 mg cholesterol; 355.8 mg sodium; 21.0 g carbohydrates; 1.8 g dietary fiber; 5.1 g protein; 103.2 mg calcium; 1.0 mg iron; 80.8 IU vitamin A; and 1.5 mg vitamin C.

Banana Split Cereal Bonanza

Have fun using different fruit preserves with this recipe. Try mango, cherry, apricot, and fig.

¼ small banana

1 tablespoon (15 g) vanilla whole-milk yogurt

2 teaspoons jam of choice

2 tablespoons (4 g) dry, low-sugar cereal

Split banana part lengthwise and place on a small plate. Cover with the yogurt and jam and sprinkle with the cereal.

YIELD: 1 toddler serving

EACH SERVING CONTAINS: 85.5 calories; 0.8 g total fat; 0.4 grams saturated fat; 2.0 mg cholesterol; 34.9 mg sodium; 19.3 g carbohydrates; 1.3 g dietary fiber; 1.3 g protein; 36.9 mg calcium; 1.3 mg iron; 135.1 IU vitamin A; and 4.7 mg vitamin C.

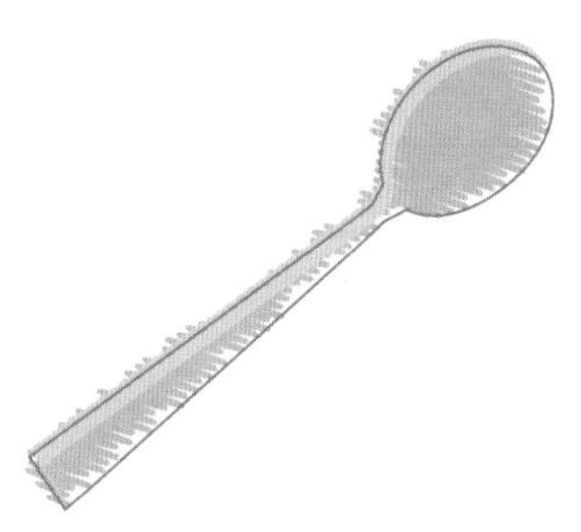

Surprising Strawberry Omelet

This is an unexpectedly delicious recipe. You can top the omelet with extra fruit for a pretty garnish.

For Omelet:

1 teaspoon butter

2 tablespoons (21 g) sliced strawberries

½ teaspoon sugar

1 egg

1 teaspoon water

For Topping:

1 tablespoon (15 g) plain yogurt

½ teaspoon sugar

STOVETOP METHOD: In a frying pan, heat the butter on low. Mix the strawberries with the sugar, and set aside. In another bowl, whisk the egg and the water and pour into the frying pan. Tilt the pan until the egg covers the whole bottom. Lift the sides of the egg with a plastic spatula and let the runny part of the egg run underneath. When the egg has cooked firmly, add the strawberries. Fold the omelet in half and press down lightly. Mix the yogurt with the sugar and add to the top of the omelet.

YIELD: 1 toddler serving

EACH SERVING CONTAINS: 135.2 calories; 8.6 g total fat; 4.5 grams saturated fat; 227.0 mg cholesterol; 72.0 mg sodium; 7.5 g carbohydrates; 0.5 g dietary fiber; 6.8 g protein; 43.5 mg calcium; 0.8 mg iron; 448.5 IU vitamin A; and 24.1 mg vitamin C.

Cuckoo for Couscous and Raisin Purée

Couscous is good in both sweet and savory dishes. Swirl in any of your toddler's favorite purées!

1/4 cup (60 ml) whole milk, plus more as desired

1/2 tablespoon (7 g) butter

2 tablespoons (20 g) plain uncooked couscous

2 tablespoons (28 g) Baby's First Raisin Purée (page 112)

STOVETOP METHOD: Bring milk and butter just to a boil in a small saucepan over medium heat. Stir in the couscous, cover, and remove from the heat. Let stand 5 minutes. Swirl in the raisin purée and add more milk as desired.

YIELD: 1 toddler serving, or scant 1/2 cup (115 g)

EACH SERVING CONTAINS: 195.7 calories; 7.9 g total fat; 5.1 grams saturated fat; 21.1 mg cholesterol; 29.2 mg sodium; 27.9 g carbohydrates; 3.2 g dietary fiber; 4.9 g protein; 74.7 mg calcium; 0.7 mg iron; 262.2 IU vitamin A; and 0.0 mg vitamin C.

Fruity Rainbow Breakfast

Feel free to substitute regular oranges for the mandarin orange segments in this recipe if those are what you have on hand. In addition to vitamin C, oranges are rich in vitamins A and B.

2 tablespoons (28 g) small curd whole-milk cottage cheese

3 mandarin orange segments (canned)

1 tablespoon (15 ml) mandarin juice

1/2 kiwi fruit

3 fresh raspberries

Place the cottage cheese in a small bowl. Finely chop the mandarin orange segments. Peel, slice, and cut kiwi into small pieces. Top cottage cheese with the orange, juice, kiwi, and raspberries.

YIELD: 1 toddler serving

EACH SERVING CONTAINS: 75.7 calories; 1.6 g total fat; 0.8 grams saturated fat; 6.3 mg cholesterol; 111.9 mg sodium; 13.0 g carbohydrates; 1.8 g dietary fiber; 3.8 g protein; 47.7 mg calcium; 0.2 mg iron; 332.1 IU vitamin A; and 46.5 mg vitamin C.

Minding Our Manners: Gentle Discipline at the Table

Toddlers at thirteen months need some freedom to experiment in order to assert their independence. Allow them to experiment with a spoon or use their fingers to try and feed themselves. However, if they start to throw food or smear it on the chair or in their hair, it's time to take it away.

To painlessly set limits about eating issues, once a child has made it clear that she is not going to eat, remove the food and take her out of the high chair. Later, when she indicates that she is hungry, either offer her the food that was removed or give her a healthy snack. Remember that we are all vulnerable to manipulation, and children are remarkably astute at using this advantage. It is important to be consistent, without being authoritarian, inflexible, punitive, or angry. All children need limits, but limits that are given with love.

Oh So Fresh Mozzarella and Tomato

Fresh mozzarella is soft, silky, and creamy, and it tastes delicious with ripe tomatoes. If you'd like, drizzle just a touch of olive oil on top of the mozzarella.

1 round slice (½-inch or 12 mm thick) fresh mozzarella cheese

1 tomato

Fresh basil leaves (optional)

Slice the tomato, place on a plate, and top with a slice of mozzarella. If you have fresh basil, cut a few leaves into pieces and place them in between the mozzarella and tomatoes.

YIELD: 1 toddler serving

EACH SERVING CONTAINS: 93.8 calories; 6.9 g total fat; 4.4 grams saturated fat; 24.9 mg cholesterol; 120.0 mg sodium; 1.6 g carbohydrates; 0.2 g dietary fiber; 6.2 g protein; 164.8 mg calcium; 0.2 mg iron; 397.8 IU vitamin A; and 4.5 mg vitamin C.

S-S-S-Smoothie!

This is a toddler recipe that the family can also enjoy. Don't be surprised if you polish off what your baby can't!

½ cup (70 g) peeled, chopped, and seeded papaya

½ banana

¼ cup (60 g) plain yogurt

1 cup (235 ml) white grape juice

2 tablespoons (28 ml) lemon juice

1 tablespoon (18 g) frozen orange juice concentrate

4 cracked ice cubes

Combine the papaya, banana, yogurt, grape juice, lemon juice, frozen orange juice concentrate, and ice cubes in a blender and blend on high 1 minute.

YIELD: 4 toddler servings, ½ cup (120 ml) each

EACH SERVING CONTAINS: 73.2 calories; 0.6 g total fat; 0.3 grams saturated fat; 2.0 mg cholesterol; 12.8 mg sodium; 17.2 g carbohydrates; 0.7 g dietary fiber; 0.9 g protein; 30.0 mg calcium; 0.1 mg iron; 217.6 IU vitamin A; and 38.1 mg vitamin C.

Unpredictable Appetites

You will likely see variations in your toddlers' appetite between one and two years of age, especially a decreased appetite. Changes in the body, changes in daily routines, and teething are some of the reasons a child's appetite may decrease. Parents often worry unduly about this, but remember that children are extremely sensitive to negative (as well as positive) emotions and will react to your anxiety. If no fuss is made over these periods of poor eating, the problem will, in all likelihood, resolve itself. However, if your child appears listless, loses weight, or continues to reject food, consult your pediatrician. A healthy child will eat when he is hungry. If food is refused, remove it after a few minutes. Don't coax, play, or use tricks to make him eat.

Wonderful Wheat Bread with Apricot Purée

This recipes also works well with Fuzzy Peach Purée (page 48) or Sweet Pear Purée (page 29).

1 slice toasted whole-wheat bread

2 teaspoons butter

1 tablespoon (15 g) Naturally Sweet Apricot Purée (page 56)

Halve the bread and spread one half with the butter and the other half with Naturally Sweet Apricot Purée. Fold the two slices together then cut into two pieces.

YIELD: 2 toddler servings, or ½ slice bread each

EACH SERVING CONTAINS: 112.9 calories; 7.8 g total fat; 5.5 grams saturated fat; 20.0 mg cholesterol; 73.2 mg sodium; 8.2 g carbohydrates; 1.3 g dietary fiber; 2.1 g protein; 17.7 mg calcium; 0.5 mg iron; 448.9 IU vitamin A; and 0.0 mg vitamin C.

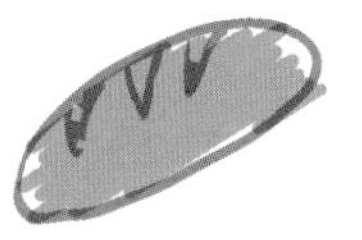

Tropical Pineapple Chiffon

This recipe can also double as "dessert." If you don't have macadamia nuts, use chopped walnuts instead.

1 tablespoon (8 g) chopped macadamia nuts

¼ cup (60 ml) pineapple juice

¼ cup (41 g) pineapple chunks (fresh or canned)

2 tablespoons (30 g) vanilla whole-milk yogurt

Process the macadamia nuts and pineapple juice in a blender until smooth. Cut pineapple chunks into small pieces. Add the yogurt and pineapple and continue to process until creamy.

YIELD: 1 toddler serving, or ½ cup (115 g)

EACH SERVING CONTAINS: 130.4 calories; 7.3 g total fat; 1.6 grams saturated fat; 4.0 mg cholesterol; 16.1 mg sodium; 15.8 g carbohydrates; 1.2 g dietary fiber; 1.9 g protein; 58.0 mg calcium; 0.4 mg iron; 78.5 IU vitamin A; and 22.3 mg vitamin C.

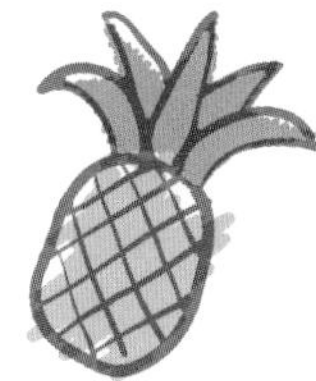

Yummy Recipe Tip: Using Fresh Pineapple

Fresh, ripe pineapple is sweeter than candy. After preparing this recipe, use the rest of the pineapple in smoothies, on salads, or as a topping for yogurt cheese or waffles.

Mini Blueberry Muffins ❄

Although this recipe calls for fresh blueberries, you can use frozen too. Add them to the batter frozen but be careful not to stir too much or the batter will turn purple. When using frozen berries, you'll have to bake the muffins 3 to 5 minutes longer.

3/4 cup (150 g) sugar

1/2 cup (115 g) plain yogurt or 1/2 cup (120 ml) buttermilk

1/4 cup (60 ml) vegetable oil

2 eggs

1 teaspoon vanilla extract

1 1/2 cups (218 g) fresh blueberries

2 cups (250 g) all-purpose flour

2 teaspoons baking soda

1/2 teaspoon salt

OVEN METHOD: Preheat the oven to 375°F (190°C, gas mark 5). Lightly grease 24 minimuffin cups. In a large bowl, mix the sugar, yogurt or buttermilk, oil, eggs, and vanilla. Fold in the blueberries. In a small bowl, combine the flour, baking soda, and salt. Blend the wet ingredients and dry ingredients together gently. Spoon the batter into prepared minimuffin cups. Bake 18 minutes until lightly golden or a cake tester inserted in center comes out clean. Remove from pan and cool on a rack.

YIELD: 12 toddler servings, or 2 minimuffins each

EACH SERVING (if using yogurt) CONTAINS: 173.2 calories; 6.0 g total fat; 1.2 grams saturated fat; 37.2 mg cholesterol; 587.0 mg sodium; 27.8 g carbohydrates; 1.0 g dietary fiber; 3.6 g protein; 87.3 mg calcium; 1.2 mg iron; 70.1 IU vitamin A; and 1.9 mg vitamin C.

Nummy Nut-Butter Kisses

This energy-packed treat is one your toddler will enjoy! Consider serving one kiss with some pear and 1/2 cup (120 ml) milk.

1/3 cup (47 g) chopped cashews

1/4 cup (65 g) smooth peanut butter

1/4 cup (32 g) dry milk powder

1 tablespoon (20 g) honey

1 teaspoon pure vanilla extract

Pulse the cashews in a blender until finely ground but not puréed. Add the peanut butter, milk powder, honey, and vanilla and pulse just until blended. With your hands, roll the peanut butter mixture into 8 little balls. (The consistency of the mixture will be soft.)

This recipe, when sealed tightly in the refrigerator, will stay fresh for up to 4 days.

YIELD: 8 toddler servings, or one "kiss" each

EACH SERVING CONTAINS: 109.6 calories; 8.0 g total fat; 2.1 grams saturated fat; 3.9 mg cholesterol; 53.4 mg sodium; 7.4 g carbohydrates; 0.7 g dietary fiber; 3.7 g protein; 39.2 mg calcium; 0.5 mg iron; 36.6 IU vitamin A; and 0.4 mg vitamin C.

Recipe Variation Tip

Substitute chopped peeled pears, peaches, or nectarines for the blueberries in this recipe for a yummy variation.

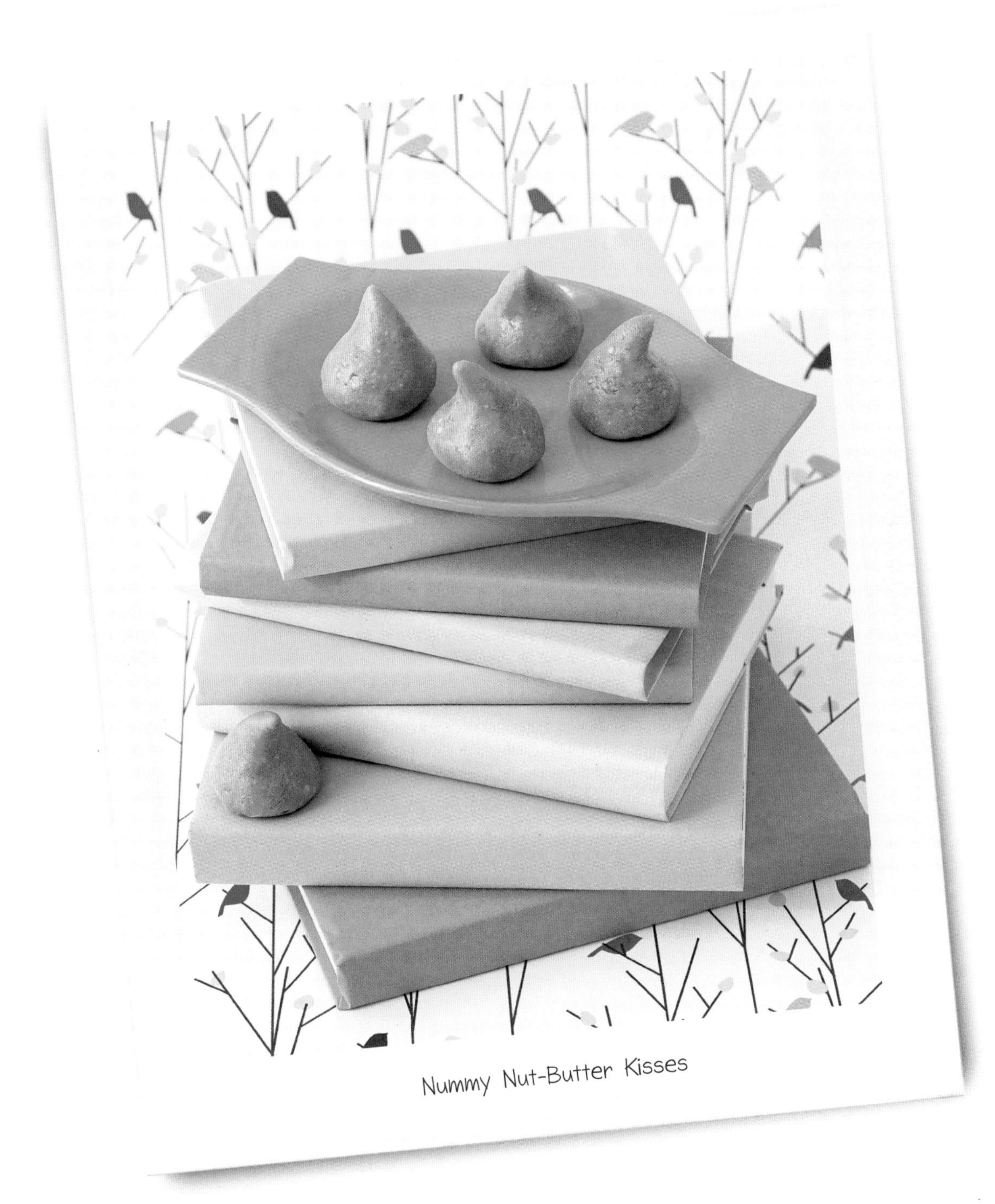

Nummy Nut-Butter Kisses

Chicken Soup and ABC Pasta

This soup is quick and easy to make. You can use raw, frozen, or cooked vegetables. If you have leftover beans, add them to the soup.

¼ cup (38 g) cooked alphabet pasta (or star, tubettini, or other small pasta)

¼ cup (about 25 g) mixed fresh or frozen vegetables, carrots, corn, peas, or green beans

¼ cup (28 g) potatoes

1 cup (235 ml) low-sodium chicken broth

⅓ cup (47 g) shredded cooked chicken

Cook pasta according to package directions. Dice vegetables. Peel, wash, cook, and cut potatoes into small pieces. Combine all ingredients in a microwave-safe bowl. Microwave for 90 seconds or until warm.

YIELD: 6 toddler servings, ½ cup (115 ml) each

EACH SERVING CONTAINS: 50.0 calories; 1.1 g total fat; 0.2 grams saturated fat; 3.4 mg cholesterol; 128.8 mg sodium; 7.6 g carbohydrates; 0.5 g dietary fiber; 2.2 g protein; 3.6 mg calcium; 0.3 mg iron; 93.5 IU vitamin A; and 1.7 mg vitamin C.

Accepting Changes in Your Toddler's Eating Patterns

During the early years, toddlers have tremendous adjustments to make and new experiences to absorb, including adapting to a large variety of foods and methods of eating. Rebellion against unfamiliar foods can be lessened and long-term refusals prevented once parents learn to recognize their child's eating habits. For example, perhaps your child takes a while to wake up in the morning and is not ready for breakfast until he's had some time to adjust to the new day. There's no reason you can't delay breakfast for a bit.

During very hot weather, appetites often diminish, so you may want to keep meals light. Here are some tips:

- Serve tuna, cheese, eggs, salads, and other dishes that are simple to prepare and eat.
- A variety of fresh fruits and vegetables will provide sufficient vitamins and minerals when supplemented with a little cereal, beans, rice, and nut butters.
- Keep fresh fruit-juice pops in your freezer for healthy and refreshing treats.
- Don't hesitate to whip up smoothies made with berries, bananas, yogurt, tofu, honey and milk.

Stelline Stars with Cottage Cheese

Stelline means "little stars" in Italian and is a favorite pasta of children worldwide. It will likely become one of your child's favorites, too! (Feel free to substitute any other small pasta if you can't find stelline, however.) Consider serving this meal with 1/4 cup (60 ml) carrot juice.

3 tablespoons (33 g) uncooked stelline (star-shaped) pasta

1 1/2 cups (355 ml) water

1 tablespoon (14 g) butter

1/4 cup (55 g) whole-fat cottage cheese

3 tablespoons cooked (28 g) fresh or (24 g) frozen green peas

STOVETOP METHOD: In a small pan, combine the pasta with the water over medium-high heat and bring to a boil. Cook 5 minutes or until the pasta is soft. Drain. Add the butter, cottage cheese, and peas. Mix well before serving.

YIELD: 2 toddler servings, 1/2 cup (115 g) each

EACH SERVING CONTAINS: 134.2 calories; 6.8 g total fat; 4.7 grams saturated fat; 20.6 mg cholesterol; 98.2 mg sodium; 12.7 g carbohydrates; 1.1 g dietary fiber; 5.1 g protein; 20.0 mg calcium; 0.6 mg iron; 313.9 IU vitamin A; and 1.0 mg vitamin C.

Awesome Avocado and Egg Sandwich

Try this sandwich filling in a mini-pita pocket for a change of pace. Just cut the pita in half so it's more manageable for little fingers.

2 teaspoons mayonnaise

1/2 slice whole wheat bread

1 slice ripe, peeled, and pitted avocado

2 slices hard-cooked egg

Spread the mayonnaise on the half slice of bread. Lightly mash the avocado and egg. Spread the mashed avocado and egg on the bread. Cut in half. Press bread slices together and cut the sandwich into small pieces or serve open-face style, cut into small pieces.

YIELD: 1 toddler serving, or 1 sandwich

EACH SERVING CONTAINS: 174.7 calories; 14.1 g total fat; 2.5 grams saturated fat; 56.5 mg cholesterol; 134.7 mg sodium; 9.5 g carbohydrates; 4.2 g dietary fiber; 3.7 g protein; 21.9 mg calcium; 0.5 mg iron; 81.2 IU vitamin A; and 2.4mg vitamin C.

Multi-Tasking Will Save You Time!

When you're preparing a meal for your family in the oven, use that opportunity to bake a potato, sweet potato, or small squash for your baby. Just scrub the vegetable, prick it with a fork, and bake it until it's tender. When it's done, let it cool, scoop out the flesh, and mix it well with breast milk or formula.

The same applies when making pasta, rice, beans, vegetables, or chicken. These are all suitable foods for a baby, so set aside plain-cooked ingredients before combining them into a family-style recipe. You'll be happy to have these on hand when your impatient toddler is hungry!

Wonderful White Bean Soup ❄

This mild tasting soup, favored by toddlers, tastes best made from scratch. If you don't have time for cooking dried beans, use canned beans. Use two 15-ounce (420 g) cans small white beans, drained, and 6 cups (1425 ml) water or four 14-ounce (425 ml) cans nonfat chicken broth.

1 cup (215 g) dried small white beans soaked overnight in 6 cups (1,425 ml) water

6 cups (1425 ml) water (for cooking)

2 bay leaves

2 tablespoons (28 ml) olive oil

1 large onion

3 large tomatoes

½ cup (30 g) fresh parsley

1 large clove garlic

1 tablespoon (15 g) kosher salt or 1 teaspoon regular salt

1 cup (105 g) uncooked small whole wheat pasta (elbow macaroni, small shells, or tubettini)

STOVETOP METHOD: Soak the beans in 6 cups (1,425 ml) of water overnight. The next day, drain and rinse the beans and place in a large saucepan with 6 cups (1425 ml) water and the bay leaves. Bring to a boil over medium heat, skim off the foam, cover, reduce the heat, and simmer 1½ hours, or until the beans are tender. Discard the bay leaves.

Heat the oil in a frying pan over medium heat. Chop the onion, add to oil, and cook, stirring occasionally, for 10 minutes. Blanch, peel, and chop the tomatoes (see tip below). Finely chop the parsley and garlic. Add the tomatoes, parsley, and garlic and cook 3 to 4 minutes.

Cook the pasta according to directions on package. Drain and add to the soup.

When the beans are tender, remove 1½ cups (273 g) beans and 1 cup (235 ml) cooking liquid and purée in a blender (or mash with a potato masher). Return the puréed beans to the saucepan; add the sautéed vegetables. Season with the salt.

YIELD: 12 toddler servings, ½ cup (120 ml) each

EACH SERVING CONTAINS: 124.4 calories; 2.9 g total fat; 0.4 grams saturated fat; 0.0 mg cholesterol; 794.6 mg sodium; 19.0 g carbohydrates; 5.1 g dietary fiber; 6.2 g protein; 49.6 mg calcium; 1.9 mg iron; 478.9 IU vitamin A; and 10.5 mg vitamin C.

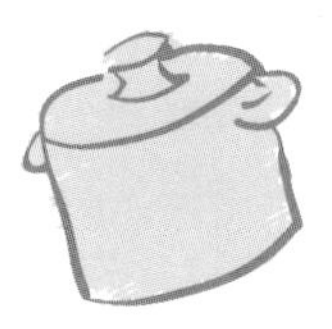

All Dressed-Up Avocado and Carrots

To easily cube the avocado, cut the flesh in a checkerboard pattern after you remove the pit, and then scoop out the avocado and the cubes will remain intact.

1 ripe avocado

1 cup (110 g) grated carrots

3 tablespoons (12 g) parsley, (3 g) cilantro or mint, finely chopped

Luscious Lime Dressing (page 143), to taste

Peel, pit, and cube the avocado. Place avocado, carrots, and parsley in a bowl and gently mix with Luscious Lime Dressing.

YIELD: 2 toddler servings, 1/2 cup (about 115 g) each

EACH SERVING (not including Luscious Lime Dressing) CONTAINS: 189.1 calories; 14.9 g total fat; 2.2 grams saturated fat; 0.0 mg cholesterol; 54.4 mg sodium; 15.1 g carbohydrates; 8.7 g dietary fiber; 2.8 g protein; 41.1 mg calcium; 1.1 mg iron; 11318.7 IU vitamin A; and 21.4 mg vitamin C.

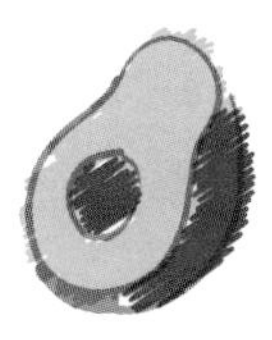

Luscious Lime Dressing

Try this lime dressing for a luscious treat.

Juice of 1 lime

1 teaspoon balsamic vinegar

2 tablespoons (28 ml) olive oil

1 teaspoon peeled and finely chopped ginger (optional)

Place lime juice, vinegar, olive oil, and ginger (if desired) in a small, clean, lidded jar and mix well.

YIELD: 4 toddler servings, 1 tablespoon (15 ml) each

EACH SERVING CONTAINS: 24.5 calories; 2.3 g total fat; 0.3 grams saturated fat; 0.0 mg cholesterol; 0.5 mg sodium; 1.o g carbohydrates; 0.0 g dietary fiber; 0.1 g protein; 1.5 mg calcium; 0.0 mg iron; 3.8 IU vitamin A; and 2.3 mg vitamin C.

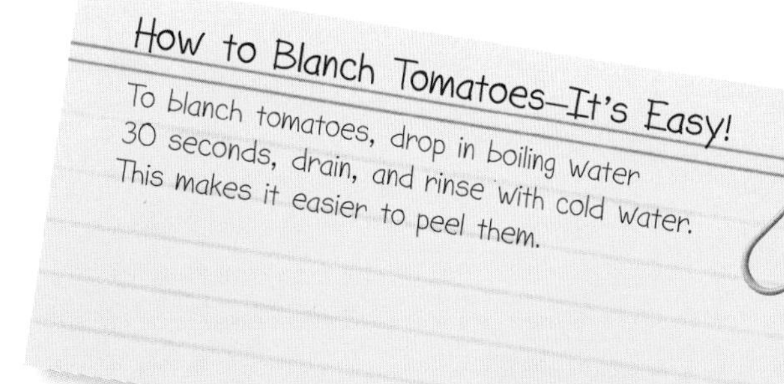

Cheesy Potato Patties

Serve these savory patties with applesauce and steamed asparagus. They also make a nice side dish for fish or chicken. Panko mix is available in the ethnic food section of most supermarkets. If you cannot find it, use Italian bread crumbs, or make your own fresh bread crumbs.

1 large (3/4 to 1 pound, or 340 to 455 g) baking potato, baked

1/2 cup (75 g) crumbled mild goat cheese

1 egg

1 tablespoon (15 ml) lemon juice

1 tablespoon (4 g) chopped fresh dill

1/2 teaspoon salt (optional)

1 cup (50 g) panko (Japanese bread crumbs)

1 tablespoon (15 ml) olive oil

1 tablespoon (14 g) butter

STOVETOP METHOD: With a spoon, scrape out all of the potato flesh from the skin and place in a medium bowl. Add the cheese and mix with a fork. In a cup, whisk the egg well with a fork and add the lemon juice, dill, and salt (if using). Add to the potato and cheese and mix thoroughly. Form into 6 patties.

Place the panko on a plate and dredge the patties, covering both sides with the crumbs. Heat the oil and butter in a frying pan over medium heat. Place the patties in the pan and fry each side 5 minutes until nicely browned. Keep turning the patties if needed to prevent burning.

YIELD: 6 toddler servings, 1 patty each

EACH SERVING CONTAINS: 203.5 calories; 9.3 g total fat; 4.9 grams saturated fat; 49.2 mg cholesterol; 105.6 mg sodium; 23.3 g carbohydrates; 2.0 g dietary fiber; 7.1 g protein; 45.7 mg calcium; 1.4 mg iron; 329.4 IU vitamin A; and 8.5 mg vitamin C.

Awesome Asparagus Soup ❄

Asparagus is an excellent source of vitamins A, C, K, and folate. Consider serving this with Italian bread.

1 1/2 pounds (680 g) fresh asparagus

3 cans (14 ounces, or 425 ml each) nonfat chicken broth or 4 cups (950 ml) homemade

1/4 cup (60 ml) olive oil

1/2 cup (80 g) chopped onion

1 cup (104 g) chopped well-washed leeks, white part only (about 2 leeks)

1/2 cup (50 g) chopped celery

1 baking potato (about 1/2 pound, or 225 g), peeled and cubed

1 tablespoon (15 ml) fresh lemon juice

Salt (to taste)

STOVETOP METHOD: Snap off asparagus tips and save. Place stalks only in a saucepan with 3 cups (700 ml) chicken broth. Bring to a boil, cover, reduce heat to low, and simmer for 45 minutes. Drain and save the broth. Discard the stalks.

Add oil to a large, heavy-bottomed pot. Add onion, leeks, celery, potato, and asparagus tips. Cover and cook on low for 40 minutes or until vegetables are soft. Add a little broth if necessary. When done, add lemon juice. Blend in two batches, along with broth. Return the soup to the saucepan, add salt to taste, and reheat. Thin soup to desired consistency by adding additional broth.

YIELD: 12 toddler servings, 1/2 cup (120 ml) each

EACH SERVING CONTAINS: 83.6 calories; 5.3 g total fat; 0.7 grams saturated fat; 0.0 mg cholesterol; 488.9 mg sodium; 7.5 g carbohydrates; 1.8 g dietary fiber; 2.4 g protein; 24.7 mg calcium; 0.9 mg iron; 739.7 IU vitamin A; and 7.9 mg vitamin C.

My Little Peanut Chicken Satay

This recipe was inspired by the classic Indonesian dish Chicken Satay. Consider serving this to your toddler with refreshing slices of cantaloupe and kiwi.

1 tablespoon (15 ml) olive oil

1 pound (455 g) ground chicken

2 tablespoons (28 ml) lime juice

¼ cup (4 g) chopped fresh cilantro

3 inner leaves romaine lettuce

1 tablespoon (15 ml) Perfect Peanut Sauce (see right)

STOVETOP METHOD: Heat the oil in a large skillet over medium heat. Add the chicken and cook 4 to 6 minutes or until cooked through. Stir in the lime juice and sprinkle with the cilantro.

To assemble, place 1 to 2 tablespoons (15 to 28 g) chicken on one lettuce leaf for your toddler and divide the remaining chicken between the two remaining leaves. Drizzle your toddler's chicken with Perfect Peanut Sauce and wrap the other pieces for later.

YIELD: 8 toddler servings, 2 ounces (55 g) each

EACH SERVING CONTAINS: 94.7 calories; 5.8 g total fat; 1.5 grams saturated fat; 48.9 mg cholesterol; 41.7 mg sodium; 0.8 g carbohydrates; 0.1 g dietary fiber; 10.2 g protein; 5.8 mg calcium; 0.6 mg iron; 43.2 IU vitamin A; and 1.5 mg vitamin C.

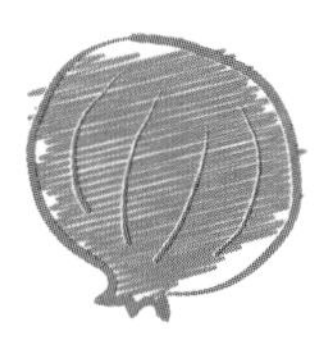

Perfect Peanut Sauce

This sauce is also good on many foods. You can refrigerate it for up to 7 days.

1 tablespoon (15 ml) olive oil

½ cup (80 g) finely chopped onion

1 clove garlic, pressed through a garlic press or minced

1 nickel-size peeled and minced piece of fresh ginger

½ cup (130 g) smooth peanut butter

2 teaspoons unpacked brown sugar

¾ to 1 cup (175 to 235 ml) water

2 teaspoons low-sodium soy sauce

STOVETOP METHOD: Heat the oil in a small saucepan over medium heat; add the onion, garlic, and ginger. Sauté 3 to 5 minutes or until the onion is soft. Add the peanut butter, brown sugar, water, and soy sauce and whisk until smooth. (It should be the consistency of pancake batter; if it's too thick, thin with a little bit more water.) Reduce heat, cover, and simmer 10 minutes or until you have the desired sauce consistency. Stir often to prevent burning. Serve at room temperature. (Oil will gather on top, so stir well before serving.)

YIELD: Sixteen one-tablespoon (15 ml) servings

EACH SERVING CONTAINS: 53.6 calories; 4.5 g total fat; 0.9 grams saturated fat; 0.0 mg cholesterol; 54.0 mg sodium; 2.6 g carbohydrates; 0.6 g dietary fiber; 1.8 g protein; 1.9 mg calcium; 0.1 mg iron; 0.0 IU vitamin A; and 0.4 mg vitamin C.

Super Quick Cup-of-Noodle Soup ❄

This soup takes five minutes to make or about the same time as preparing the commercial brand. You can omit the green onion, if you wish.

1 can (14 ounces, or 425 ml) low-sodium chicken broth (or 1½ cups, or 355 ml homemade)

1 baby carrot

1 piece (3 inches, or 7.5 cm) green onion

2 tablespoons (20 g) frozen corn or 1 tablespoon (10 g) each frozen corn and peas

1 ounce (about ¾ cup, or 15 g) egg noodles

½ teaspoon tamari (natural soy sauce) or light soy sauce (optional)

STOVETOP METHOD: Bring the broth to a boil in a small pan over medium-high heat. Shred the baby carrot and thinly slice the green onion. Add the carrot, green onion, and corn to the broth and cook 2 minutes. Add the noodles and cook 3 more minutes. Season with soy sauce if desired.

YIELD: 5 toddler servings, ½ cup (120 ml) each

EACH SERVING (not including soy sauce) CONTAINS: 23.5 calories; 0.5 g total fat; 0.0 grams saturated fat; 3.1 mg cholesterol; 363.1 mg sodium; 3.5 g carbohydrates; 0.4 g dietary fiber; 1.1 g protein; 3.1 mg calcium; 0.1 mg iron; 381.9 IU vitamin A; and 0.8 mg vitamin C.

Toddler's Shepherd's Pie

If you're making a turkey meatloaf or turkey burgers for your family, this is a wonderful dish to serve your toddler. Just set aside some ground turkey before you season the meat.

¼ cup (80 g) cooked ground turkey

¼ cup (56 g) cooked mashed potatoes

2 tablespoons (15 g) grated Cheddar cheese

OVEN METHOD: Preheat the oven to 350°F (180°C, gas mark 4). Lightly oil an oven-safe 6-ounce (175 ml) custard cup. Place the turkey in the cup, cover with the potatoes, and sprinkle with the cheese. Bake 10 to 15 minutes until the cheese is melted.

MICROWAVE METHOD: Lightly oil a microwave-safe custard cup. Place the turkey in the cup, cover with the potatoes, and sprinkle with the cheese. Microwave on high 30 to 60 seconds until the cheese has melted and the pie is heated through.

YIELD: 1 toddler serving

EACH SERVING CONTAINS: 251.8 calories; 11.6 g total fat; 3.2 grams saturated fat; 84.1 mg cholesterol; 338.1 mg sodium; 8.6 g carbohydrates; 1.2 g dietary fiber; 26.6 g protein; 70.0 mg calcium; 1.5 mg iron; 100.0 IU vitamin A; and 0.0 mg vitamin C.

Let Your Child Experiment with Hand Preference

Left- or right-handed dominance has not yet been established at sixteen months and should not be enforced. Allow your child to grab the spoon with either hand. In another three or four months, handedness will probably be evident, and finer control of the wrist and fingers will be established, so self-feeding will be considerably more efficient and speedy.

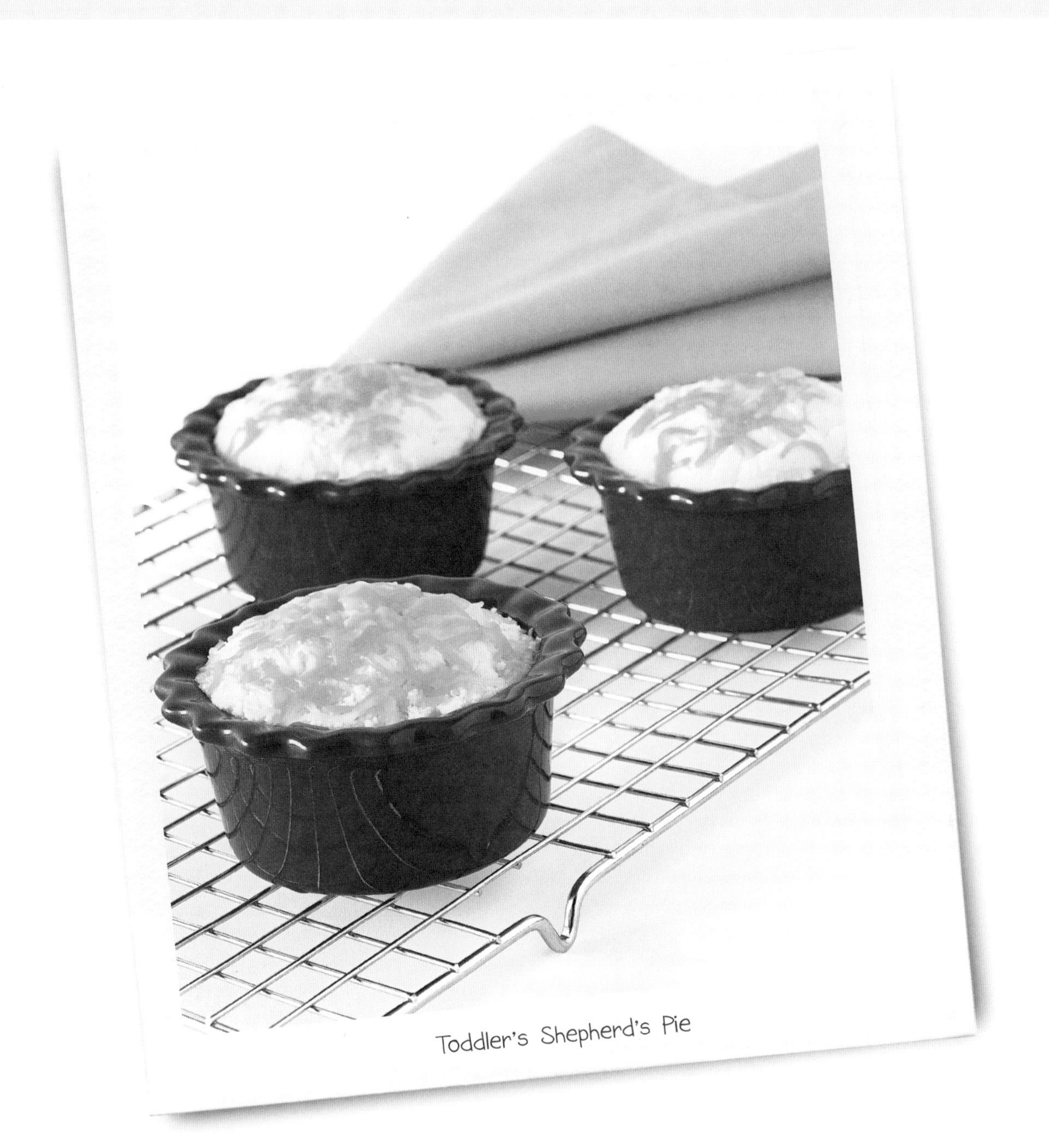

Toddler's Shepherd's Pie

All Grown Up Chicken with Rice and Broccoli

Consider serving this recipe with fresh raspberries with a splash of milk.

1 boneless, skinless chicken tender

1 broccoli floret

2 tablespoons (21 g) cooked rice

MICROWAVE METHOD: Cook the chicken tender according to package directions. Microwave the broccoli until cooked through. Chop the chicken and broccoli into small pieces. Serve with the rice.

YIELD: 1 toddler serving

EACH SERVING CONTAINS: 215.5 calories; 10.2 g total fat; 2.2 grams saturated fat; 25.0 mg cholesterol; 865.4 mg sodium; 17.9 g carbohydrates; 1.4 g dietary fiber; 12.1 g protein; 31.0 mg calcium; 1.4 mg iron; 498.2 IU vitamin A; and 3.8 mg vitamin C.

Lentils and Rice with Yogurt Sauce

If you have some lentils already cooked, a bit of leftover rice, and tomato sauce (homemade or store-bought), you can put together this complete and tasty meal for your toddler in a couple of minutes. Consider serving with 1⁄4 cup (60 ml) milk and some banana for dessert.

1 tablespoon (12 g) cooked lentils

1 tablespoon (10 g) cooked rice

2 tablespoons (28 g) homemade or store-bought tomato sauce

1 tablespoon (15 g) plain yogurt

MICROWAVE METHOD: Combine the lentils, rice, and tomato sauce in a small cup. Microwave on high 30 seconds. Stir in the yogurt. Allow to cool slightly before serving.

YIELD: 1 toddler serving

EACH SERVING CONTAINS: 43.6 calories; 0.6 g total fat; 0.3 grams saturated fat; 2.0 mg cholesterol; 167.4 mg sodium; 7.9 g carbohydrates; 1.5 g dietary fiber; 2.4 g protein; 21.8 mg calcium; 0.7 mg iron; 166.1 IU vitamin A; and 3.3 mg vitamin C.

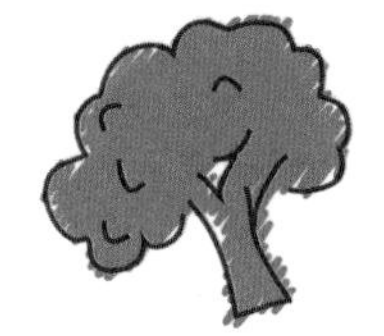

Out on the Town with Toddlers

Taking small children shopping is usually done out of necessity, not choice. Little ones get bored and restless easily, and by the time parents decide to stop for a snack or lunch, toddlers are often too tired to eat. One of the most common reasons for poor appetite is fatigue. Sitting in a chair for any length of time is also very trying for a child.

What to do? Look for alternatives to going to restaurants and coffee shops. If the weather is nice, find a park, small grassy area, or even a bench and have a mini-picnic. Either bring food from home, or buy healthy restaurant food. Assorted cheese and crackers or small sandwiches, fresh fruit, milk, or juice packed in a little ice chest are perfect for a shopping lunch. If you feel like restaurant food, many venues have take-out.

As your toddler grows, you'll be able to share restaurant meals. A bigger concern will be how to keep your little one entertained while waiting for food. A story, simple puzzle, or a couple of favorite toys usually keep a toddler occupied, but your attention and participation will be needed. Expecting a small child to entertain herself for a long period of time is unreasonable.

Baby Sliders ❄

Consider serving this dish with boiled, mashed, or baked potatoes or carrots. For dessert, serve a piece of peeled watermelon with the seeds removed.

1 egg

2 tablespoons (28 ml) whole milk

½ pound (225 g) ground beef

2 tablespoons (14 g) plain bread crumbs

2 teaspoons olive oil

STOVETOP METHOD: Whisk the egg and milk together in a small cup. In a medium bowl, mix the ground beef with the bread crumbs. Add the egg mixture and mix. With your hands, form the meat into 4 small cakes.

Heat the oil in a frying pan over medium heat. Add the cakes and cook, turning often, until the cakes are cooked through and a meat thermometer inserted sideways into the patties registers 165°F (74°C).

The meat cakes can be refrigerated, covered, for 2 to 3 days. You can also freeze them, individually wrapped with plastic wrap, for up to 2 months.

YIELD: 4 toddler servings, or one 2-ounce (55 g) meat cake each

EACH SERVING CONTAINS: 221.6 calories; 18.0 g total fat; 6.2 grams saturated fat; 96.7 mg cholesterol; 84.5 mg sodium; 3.0 g carbohydrates; 0.1 g dietary fiber; 11.1 g protein; 30.4 mg calcium; 1.4 mg iron; 82.8 IU vitamin A; and 0 mg vitamin C.

Toddler's First Tuna Casserole

Tuna is a high-quality source of protein and is a good source of heart-healthy omega-3 fatty acids. This is a quick, tasty, and easy meal.

½ can (5.4 ounces, or 160 ml) cream of mushroom soup (low salt), undiluted

1 cup (140 g) cooked whole wheat farfalle pasta (also called bow tie or butterfly pasta)

1 can (5 ounces, or 140 g) chunk light tuna, packed in water

¼ cup (38 g) fresh or (33 g) frozen peas

¼ cup (60 ml) whole milk

MICROWAVE METHOD: Stir the soup into the pasta and mix well. Add the tuna, peas, and milk. Cover and microwave on high 3 minutes, stirring halfway through, until the casserole is thoroughly heated.

YIELD: 4 toddler servings, ½ cup (about 115 g) each

EACH SERVING CONTAINS: 122.3 calories; 2.5 g total fat; 0.8 grams saturated fat; 21.6 mg cholesterol; 175.0 mg sodium; 13.5 g carbohydrates; 1.7 g dietary fiber; 11.2 g protein; 27.6 mg calcium; 0.5 mg iron; 54.0 IU vitamin A; and 0.6 mg vitamin C.

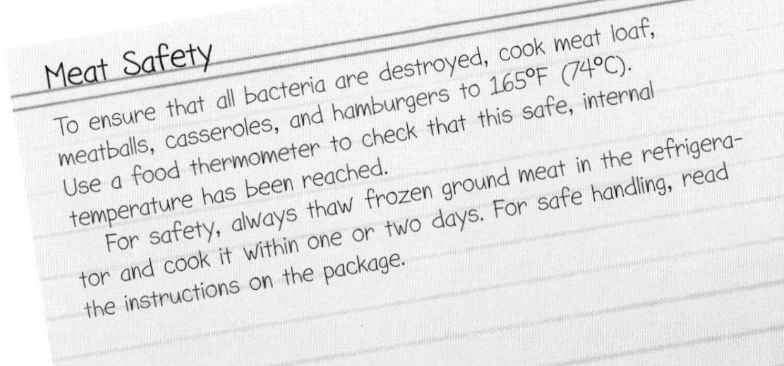

Meat Safety

To ensure that all bacteria are destroyed, cook meat loaf, meatballs, casseroles, and hamburgers to 165°F (74°C). Use a food thermometer to check that this safe, internal temperature has been reached.

For safety, always thaw frozen ground meat in the refrigerator and cook it within one or two days. For safe handling, read the instructions on the package.

Bok Bok Chicken, Noodles, and Carrots

As simple as these ingredients are, toddlers (and adults!) never seem to tire of this classic combination. Plus, it's fun to eat and healthy!

1 small boneless, skinless chicken tender (about 2 ounces, or 55 g)

2 baby carrots

1/4 cup (40 g) cooked egg noodles

2 teaspoons butter

MICROWAVE METHOD: Cook the chicken tender according to package instructions and shred into bite-size pieces. Cut the carrots into thin sticks and put in a microwave-safe bowl with a little water and cook 90 seconds or until tender. Mix chicken, cooked egg noodles, and carrots together, top with butter, and microwave 20 seconds or until ingredients are warmed through. Serve as finger food.

Leftovers can be safely refrigerated in a covered container for 3 to 4 days.

YIELD: 3 toddler servings (1 tender each)

EACH SERVING CONTAINS: 193.5 calories; 10.1 g total fat; 2.2 grams saturated fat; 25.0 mg cholesterol; 269.2 mg sodium; 15.2 g carbohydrates; 1.4 g dietary fiber; 9.9 g protein; 15.5 mg calcium; 0.8 mg iron; 2779.4 IU vitamin A; and 1.3mg vitamin C.

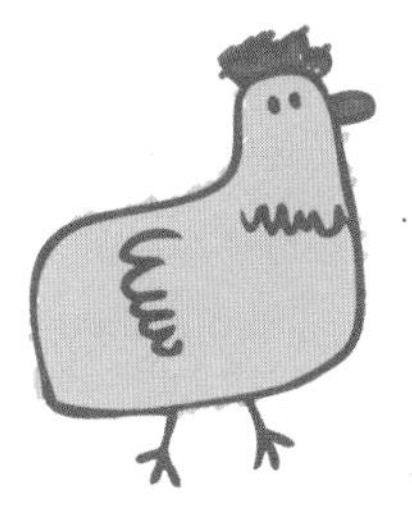

Flaky, Fantastic Fish Sticks

The tempura and panko in these fish sticks make them light and crunchy on the outside and flaky on the inside. Consider serving with Better-for-Baby Sweet Potato Fries (page 60), green beans, and watermelon (rind and seeds removed) for dessert.

1 pound (455 g) fresh or frozen boneless skinless cod

1/2 cup (115 g) Tempura Batter Mix

1 egg

1/4 cup (60 ml) milk

1/2 cup (25 g) panko or (60 g) regular bread crumbs

1 tablespoon (15 ml) olive oil

OVEN AND STOVETOP METHODS: Preheat the oven to 475°F (240°C, gas mark 9). Cut the fish into 8 even stick-shaped pieces. Make absolutely sure that every bone has been removed from the fish.

Place the tempura batter mix on one plate. Whisk the egg and milk together in a small, shallow bowl. Place the panko on a second plate. Coat the fish sticks first in the tempura batter mix, dip in the egg-milk mix, and then coat with the panko.

Heat 1 tablespoon (15 ml) of the oil in a frying pan over medium heat. Place the fish sticks in the frying pan and cook the fish 1 minute on each side. Transfer the fish to an ovenproof baking dish. Bake 5 minutes until the fish is cooked through.

YIELD: 8 toddler servings, or one 2-ounce (55 g) fish stick each

EACH SERVING CONTAINS: 115.0 calories; 3.0 g total fat; 0.7 grams saturated fat; 52.0 mg cholesterol; 89.6 mg sodium; 8.5 g carbohydrates; 0.1 g dietary fiber; 11.8 g protein; 21.2 mg calcium; 0.4 mg iron; 68.0 IU vitamin A; and 0.6 mg vitamin C.

Perfect Poached Cod

Serve this with boiled, baked, or microwaved potato and cooked spinach. Other fish that may be prepared this way include haddock and sole.

2 ounces (55 g) cod fillet (fresh or frozen), skin and bones removed

1 small carrot

3-inch (7.5 cm) piece celery

1/4 cup (60 ml) water

1 tablespoon (14 g) butter

STOVETOP METHOD: Remove the skin and bones from the fish. Slice the carrot and celery. Place the fish, carrot, celery, and water in a small pan. Slowly bring to a simmer and cook 5 minutes. Lightly mash the fish, carrots, and celery together and top with butter.

YIELD: 1 toddler serving

EACH SERVING CONTAINS: 160.8 calories; 11.4 g total fat; 11.4 grams saturated fat; 54.4 mg cholesterol; 50.7 mg sodium; 3.2 g carbohydrates; 0.8 g dietary fiber; 10.5 g protein; 18.3 mg calcium; 0.2 mg iron; 4620.1 IU vitamin A; and 2.8 mg vitamin C.

To-riffic Tofu with Veggies and Peanut Sauce

Tofu takes on the flavor of whatever it's cooked with. Here, the sauce gives the tofu a nice, nutty flavor.

1 teaspoon olive oil

1 small slice extra firm tofu

1 baby carrot

1 small broccoli floret

1 small cauliflower floret

1 tablespoon (15 ml) Perfect Peanut Sauce (page 145), warmed

STOVETOP METHOD: Heat the oil in a small frying pan over medium heat. Add the tofu and cook until nicely browned. Turn the tofu and brown the other side. Cut into small pieces.

Place the carrot, broccoli, and cauliflower in a small steamer basket. Place the basket in a pot with 1 inch (2.5 cm) of boiling water. Cover and steam 3 to 5 minutes, until tender. Cut the carrot diagonally in half.

Assemble a plate with the broccoli, cauliflower, carrot, and tofu, and drizzle with the peanut sauce. Or place the peanut sauce on the side and let your toddler use it as dipping sauce.

YIELD: 1 toddler serving

EACH SERVING CONTAINS: 155.3 calories; 10.8 g total fat; 1.8 grams saturated fat; 0.0 mg cholesterol; 120.7 mg sodium; 6.9 g carbohydrates; 1.6 g dietary fiber; 8.6 g protein; 36.5 mg calcium; 1.2 mg iron; 285.0 IU vitamin A; and 11.0 mg vitamin C.

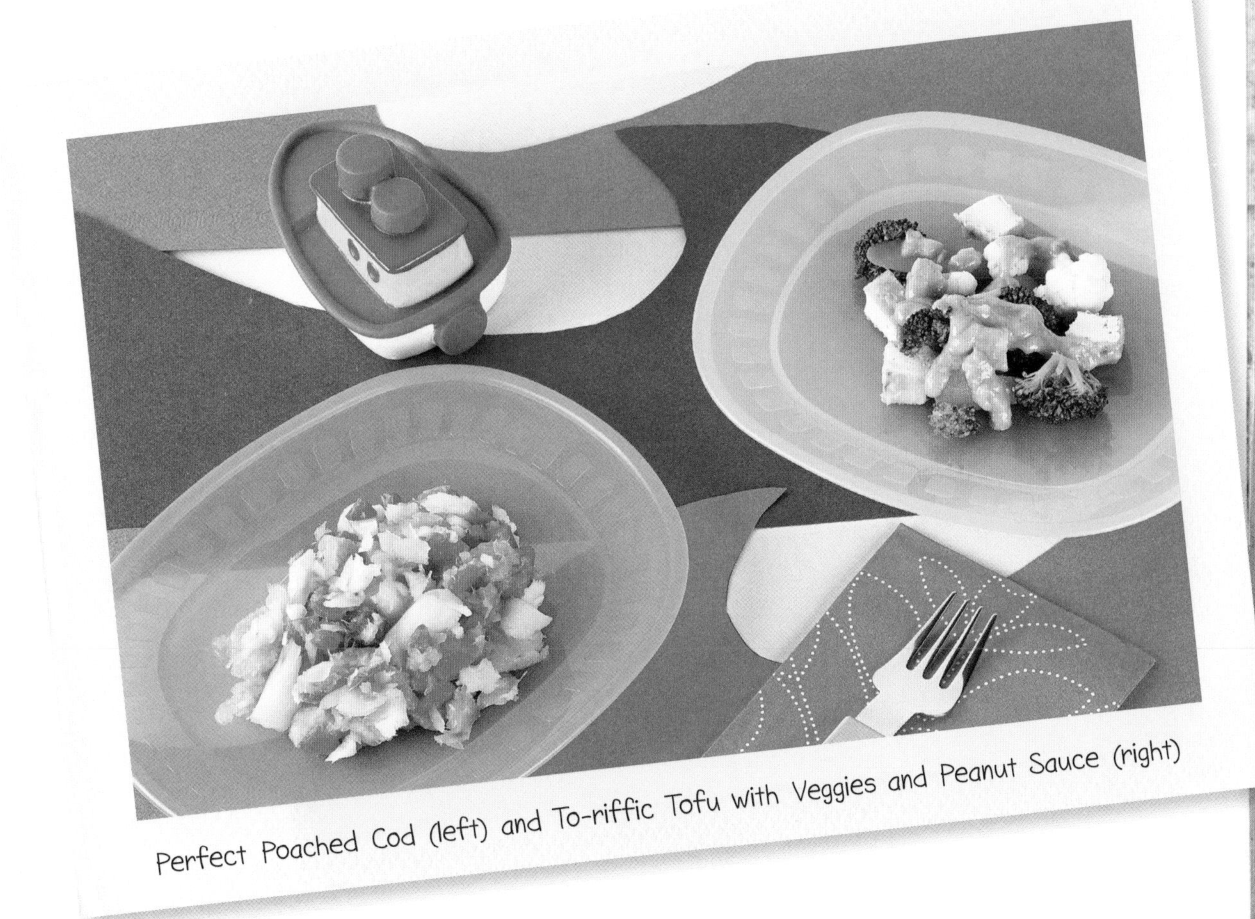

Perfect Poached Cod (left) and To-riffic Tofu with Veggies and Peanut Sauce (right)

Marvelous Macaroni-Broccoli Sauté

If your toddler doesn't like the taste of garlic, just omit it. This dish tastes even better when you serve your toddler's favorite flavor of sorbet for dessert!

1 tablespoon (15 ml) olive oil

1 teaspoon minced garlic

1/4 cup (45 g) finely diced tomatoes

3/4 cup (abut 153 g) steamed and chopped broccoli

1/4 cup (35 g) cooked whole wheat elbow macaroni

STOVETOP METHOD: Heat the oil in a heavy-bottomed pan over medium heat. Add the garlic and sauté 30 seconds. Add the tomatoes and sauté 3 minutes. Add the broccoli and sauté 2 minutes more. Reduce the heat to low and add the macaroni. Stir to blend well and simmer until heated through.

YIELD: 5 toddler servings, 1/4 cup (about 55 g) each

EACH SERVING CONTAINS: 49.5 calories; 3.0 g total fat; 0.4 grams saturated fat; 0.0 mg cholesterol; 29.6 mg sodium; 4.5 g carbohydrates; 1.0 g dietary fiber; 1.3 g protein; 20.4 mg calcium; 0.4 mg iron; 196.8 IU vitamin A; and 26.8 mg vitamin C.

Benjamin Bunny's Carrot Purée

Carrots are among children's favorite vegetables. They're considered a rich antioxidant food and one that promotes good vision and helps prevent disease.

1/2 cup (55 g) shredded baby carrots

1/4 cup (60 ml) water

1/2 tablespoon (7 g) butter

2 tablespoons (28 ml) warm whole milk

1 tablespoon (5 g) finely-grated Parmesan cheese

MICROWAVE METHOD: Place carrots and water in a small microwave-safe dish. Cover and microwave on high for 3 minutes or until carrots are soft. Drain carrots and transfer to blender. Add butter, milk, and grated cheese. Blend well, scraping down sides of blender as needed.

YIELD: 1 toddler serving, or 1/4 cup (about 55 grams)

EACH SERVING CONTAINS: 125.0 calories; 8.7 g total fat; 6.07 grams saturated fat; 6.1 mg cholesterol; 170.0 mg sodium; 7.4 g carbohydrates; 1.3 g dietary fiber; 4.7 g protein; 137.8 mg calcium; 0.0 mg iron; 8564.4 IU vitamin A; and 4.0mg vitamin C.

Toddler's Favorite Teriyaki Chicken ❄

This dish is very quick to make, and it's a toddler favorite. Serve with basmati or brown rice and steamed asparagus, a green salad, and fresh fruit for dessert.

4 ounces (115 g) boneless, skinless chicken tenders

2 tablespoons (28 ml) low-salt teriyaki sauce

OVEN METHOD: Place the chicken between two sheets of plastic wrap; with a mallet, pound lightly to an even thickness. Cut the chicken into 1-inch (2.5 cm) wide strips. Place the chicken in a bowl and add the teriyaki sauce; toss to evenly coat the chicken. Marinate 5 to 7 minutes in the refrigerator.

Preheat the broiler. Spray a broiler pan with nonstick cooking spray. Arrange the chicken strips in a single layer on the broiler pan. Broil 2 to 3 minutes on each side or until cooked through. Finely chop 1 or 2 strips for your toddler.

YIELD: 2 toddler servings, 2 ounces (55 g) each

EACH SERVING CONTAINS: 176.1 calories; 10.0 g total fat; 2.2 grams saturated fat; 25.0 mg cholesterol; 519.1 mg sodium; 11.6 g carbohydrates; 0.7 g dietary fiber; 9.0 g protein; 12.0 mg calcium; 0.7 mg iron; 0.0 IU vitamin A; and 0.4 mg vitamin C.

Tasty Tubettini with Peas

This is a quick dish to make when your tot is hungry and can't wait for dinner. Substitute any of your little one's favorite vegetables for the peas, if you wish. If you have some fresh or defrosted ground beef or turkey, fry up a couple of tablespoons and add to the pasta.

4 cups (950 ml) water

1/4 cup (25 g) uncooked whole wheat tubettini pasta

1/4 cup (33 g) frozen petite peas

2 teaspoons olive oil

2 tablespoons (10 g) grated Parmesan cheese

STOVETOP METHOD: Bring the water to a boil. Add the pasta and cook 5 minutes. Add the peas and cook 5 minutes more until pasta is just tender and peas are heated through. Drain the pasta and peas and place in small bowl. Stir in the oil and cheese.

YIELD: 1 toddler serving

EACH SERVING CONTAINS: 263.9 calories; 14.5 g total fat; 4.3 grams saturated fat; 15.0 mg cholesterol; 259.5 mg sodium; 23.2 g carbohydrates; 3.7 g dietary fiber; 10.6 g protein; 188.9 mg calcium; 1.1 mg iron; 149.3 IU vitamin A; and 2.2 mg vitamin C.

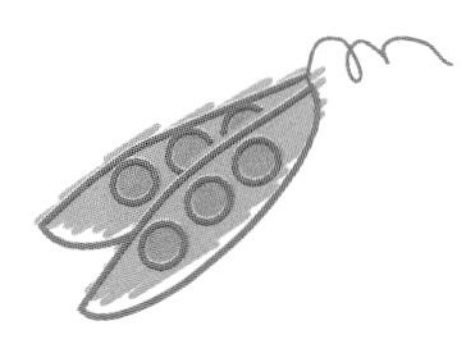

WATCH ME, MOM! MEALS FOR THE ACTIVE TODDLER:

RECIPES FOR EIGHTEEN TO TWENTY-THREE MONTHS

At eighteen months, your toddler's eating habits may be very erratic. She may eat a lot at one meal and nothing at another. She may want to eat the same food over and over again and then, one day, suddenly refuse to eat it at all. It can be a difficult time, but never force food or make a big issue out of it. If your toddler continues to grow and stays healthy, she is getting adequate nutrition. During these months, continue to give your toddler cereals, whole milk, and whole-milk dairy products. Your toddler still needs three small meals, plus one morning and one afternoon snack.

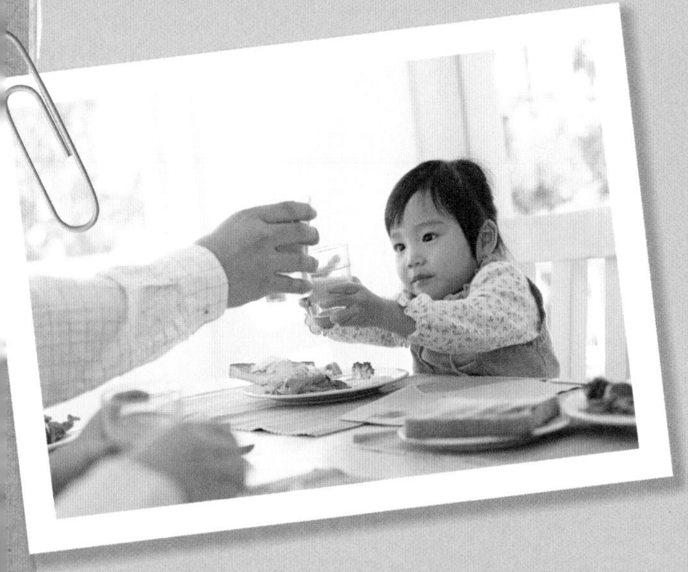

Summer Fruit Delight

This fruit mix is high in vitamin C. To turn the recipe into a smoothie, pour all ingredients into a blender and mix, adding a bit of pineapple or orange juice to thin.

2 tablespoons (20 g) cubed ripe melon

2 tablespoons (20 g) cubed fresh pineapple

2 tablespoons (20 g) diced ripe pears

1/4 small banana, sliced

1 tablespoon (18 g) frozen orange juice concentrate

Combine the melon, pineapple, pears, banana, and frozen orange juice in a bowl and toss. Chill at least 1 hour before serving. Lightly mash the fruit for your toddler and serve.

YIELD: 1 toddler serving, or 1/2 cup (about 115 g)

EACH SERVING CONTAINS: 82.5 calories; 0.2 g total fat; 0.1 grams saturated fat; 0.0 mg cholesterol; 3.9 mg sodium; 20.9 g carbohydrates; 1.9 g dietary fiber; 0.9 g protein; 7.8 mg calcium; 0.2 mg iron; 711.9 IU vitamin A; and 40.1 mg vitamin C.

My First Avocado and Cheddar Omelet

You can prepare this omelet with other mild-tasting cheeses such as mozzarella or jack too.

1 teaspoon butter

1 egg

1 teaspoon water

2 tablespoons (29 g) mashed avocado

1 heaping tablespoon (15 g) shredded Cheddar cheese

1 tablespoon (15 g) yogurt cheese (page 104) or light sour cream

STOVETOP METHOD: Melt the butter in a frying pan over medium heat. Whisk the egg and water vigorously with a fork and pour into the pan. Rotate the pan until the egg covers the whole bottom of the pan. With a rubber spatula, move the cooked egg toward the middle of the pan and let the uncooked egg spread to the sides. Continue to cook, moving the cooked egg toward the center, until the egg is almost set. Spoon the avocado and cheese on top. Fold the omelet in half and continue to cook until the cheese has melted. Cut into small pieces, and top with yogurt cheese or sour cream.

YIELD: 1 toddler serving, or one omelet

EACH SERVING (if using light sour cream) CONTAINS: 181.8 calories; 14.0 g total fat; 5.8 grams saturated fat; 231.2 mg cholesterol; 132.0 mg sodium; 4.7 g carbohydrates; 2.2 g dietary fiber; 9.6 g protein; 78.5 mg calcium; 0.9 mg iron; 625.3 IU vitamin A; and 2.9 mg vitamin C.

Pretty Please Pear Omelet

This recipe works best with a very ripe pear.

1 teaspoon butter

1 egg

1 teaspoon water

¼ cup (40 g) peeled and chopped pear

1 tablespoon (15 g) yogurt cheese (page 104)

STOVETOP METHOD: Melt the butter in a small frying pan over low heat. Whisk the egg with the water and pour into the pan. Cook, turning once, until the egg is well set. Add the pear and fold the omelet in half. Top the omelet with yogurt cheese.

YIELD: 1 toddler serving, or one omelet

EACH SERVING CONTAINS: 138.0 calories; 8.2 g total fat; 4.2 grams saturated fat; 225.5 mg cholesterol; 76.8 mg sodium; 8.7 g carbohydrates; 1.2 g dietary fiber; 7.3 g protein; 53.5 mg calcium; 0.8 mg iron; 443.6 IU vitamin A; and 1.8 mg vitamin C.

Perfectly Plain Granola

This is a granola that works well for toddlers because it doesn't contain nuts, raisins, or pieces of dried fruit, which can be choking hazards. Serve this plain or with plain yogurt topped with your favorite fresh fruit and berries. Use old-fashioned rolled oats for best results.

4 cups (320 g) old-fashioned rolled oats

⅓ cup (80 ml) maple syrup

⅓ cup (80 ml) olive oil

¼ teaspoon salt

OVEN AND STOVETOP METHOD: Preheat oven to 325°F (170°C, gas mark 3). Place the oats in a large bowl. Combine the syrup, oil, and salt in a small pan and heat over medium a few minutes until warmed through. Do not let mixture boil. Add to the oats and stir until completely blended.

Spread mixture on an 11 x 17-inch (28 x 43 cm) baking sheet. Bake on the middle rack for 15 to 20 minutes, stirring and re-spreading every 5 minutes, until the oats have turned golden.

Cool completely before you store the granola in an airtight container. It will keep at room temperature for up to 4 weeks.

YIELD: 14 toddler servings, ¼ cup (55 g) each

EACH SERVING CONTAINS: 173.2 calories; 7.2 g total fat; 1.1 grams saturated fat; 0.2 mg cholesterol; 1.1 mg sodium; 23.0 g carbohydrates; 3.0 g dietary fiber; 3.6 g protein; 14.8 mg calcium; 1.2 mg iron; 2.4 IU vitamin A; and 0.0 mg vitamin C.

Aussie Smoothie

Since the macadamia is native to Australia, this recipe is a tribute to Australians. Macadamia nuts are high in protein and fiber and are a healthy source of energy to keep your toddler going strong.

1 tablespoon (8 g) chopped macadamia nuts

¼ cup (60 ml) orange juice

1 kiwi fruit

2 tablespoons (30 g) vanilla whole-milk yogurt

Combine the nuts and juice in a blender and purée. Peel and cut the kiwi into small pieces. Add the kiwi and yogurt to the blender and process until smooth.

YIELD: 1 toddler serving

EACH SERVING CONTAINS: 150.0 calories; 7.5 g total fat; 1.6 grams saturated fat; 4.0 mg cholesterol; 79.2 mg sodium; 19.6 g carbohydrates; 3.2 g dietary fiber; 3.3 g protein; 68.5 mg calcium; 0.5 mg iron; 158.9 IU vitamin A; and 102.2 mg vitamin C.

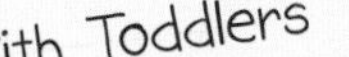

Eating on the Go with Toddlers

Taking toddlers on a trip can be an enjoyable and memorable experience. Without careful planning, however, it may be less than pleasant! Here are some food-related tips for traveling with a little one:

- Bring individual bags of simple foods that will not spoil, are easy to eat, and are enjoyed by your child. Fruits and cooked vegetables, hard cheeses, and crackers or toast are good choices.
- Consider taking along a small insulated bag to keep cheeses and fruits chilled. Instead of ice packs, freeze juice boxes or small bottles of water and use them to keep your foods cold. The bonus is that you'll have more beverages to offer your toddler when the drinks defrost!
- Keep juice and milk in a thermos. Pre-frozen cartons of juice are welcome when the weather is very warm.
- When flying, changes in air pressure can wreak havoc on little ears. Swallowing during cabin-pressure changes minimizes the possibility of earaches or other discomforts. Be sure to keep several bottles of formula, and water handy for takeoffs and landings.

Happy Hot Wheat Cereal

You may want to serve this cereal with a dot of butter and a little milk.

½ cup (120 ml) whole milk

1½ tablespoons (15 g) wheat cereal

MICROWAVE METHOD: Combine the milk and wheat cereal in a large microwave-safe bowl. Microwave on high 1 minute. Stir. Microwave 1 or 2 minutes more until the cereal thickens, stirring every 30 seconds. Watch carefully to prevent boiling over. Stir and let stand until cereal is the desired consistency and cool enough to eat.

STOVETOP METHOD: In a small saucepan, heat the milk to boiling, stirring and watching that the milk doesn't boil over. Gradually stir in cereal and bring to a boil. Reduce the heat and cook 2½ minutes or until it has thickened, stirring continuously. Let stand until the cereal is cool enough to eat.

YIELD: 1 toddler serving, or ½ cup (115 g)

EACH SERVING CONTAINS: 127.7 calories; 4.0 g total fat; 2.3 grams saturated fat; 12.2 mg cholesterol; 48.8 mg sodium; 16.9 g carbohydrates; 0.5 g dietary fiber; 5.3 g protein; 228.8 mg calcium; 4.1 mg iron; 124.4 IU vitamin A; and 0.0 mg vitamin C.

Little Stars and Raisins

This dish can be served plain or with milk and fruit. The plain pasta is also good topped with 1 tablespoon (15 g) applesauce or Naturally Sweet Apricot Purée (page 56).

1 cup (235 ml) water

3 tablespoons (12 g) uncooked stelline (star-shaped) pasta

1 tablespoon (9 g) raisins

¼ cup (60 ml) whole milk

Fruit of choice

STOVETOP METHOD: Bring the water to a boil in a saucepan over medium-high heat. Add the pasta and raisins. Simmer, uncovered and stirring occasionally, 10 minutes until the pasta is just tender. Drain. Add the milk and fruit of choice.

YIELD: 1 toddler serving, or ½ cup (115 g)

EACH SERVING (not including fruit of choice) CONTAINS: 121.9 calories; 2.2 g total fat; 1.2 grams saturated fat; 6.1 mg cholesterol; 27.8 mg sodium; 21.6 g carbohydrates; 1.5 g dietary fiber; 4.0 g protein; 80.6 mg calcium; 0.8 mg iron; 66.2 IU vitamin A; and 16.8 mg vitamin C.

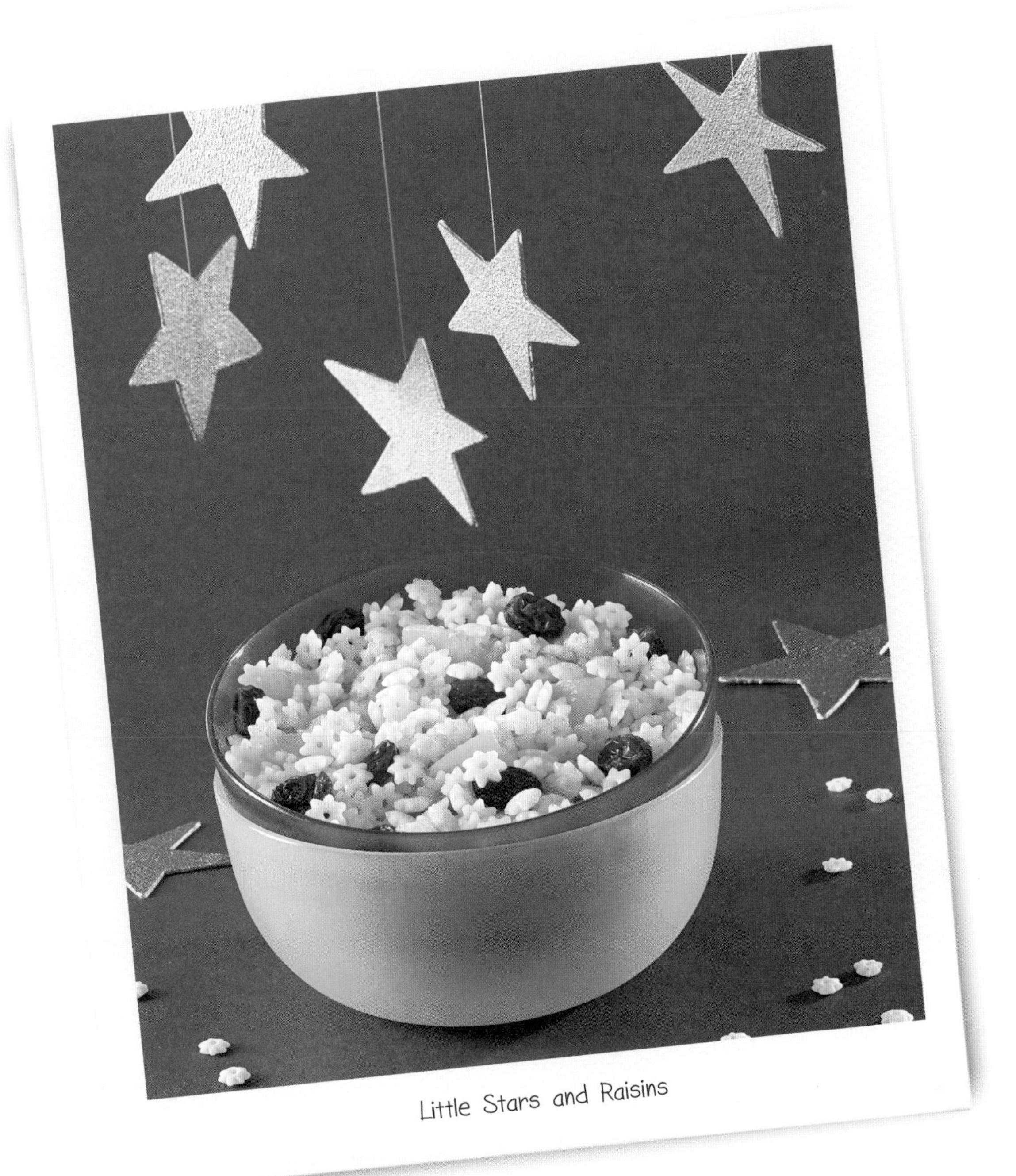

Little Stars and Raisins

Wonderfully Warm Grapefruit Crunch

Grapefruit delivers lots of nutritional goodness in the form of vitamins A and C and potassium.

1/4 sweet grapefruit

Sprinkle of brown sugar or honey

1 tablespoon (15 g) full-fat cottage cheese

1 tablespoon (7 g) nutty wheat cereal

MICROWAVE METHOD: Segment the grapefruit, place in a microwave-safe bowl, and sprinkle with the brown sugar or honey. Microwave on high 10 seconds, or until the sugar is melted. Cool, top with the cottage cheese, and sprinkle with wheat cereal.

YIELD: 1 toddler serving

EACH SERVING (if using honey) CONTAINS: 81.0 calories; 0.7 g total fat; 0.4 grams saturated fat; 3.1 mg cholesterol; 85.8 mg sodium; 17.2 g carbohydrates; 1.1 g dietary fiber; 2.3 g protein; 19.6 mg calcium; 0.5 mg iron; 348.4 IU vitamin A; and 22.8 mg vitamin C.

How to Segment a Grapefruit

To segment a grapefruit:

1. Cut the fruit in half.
2. Using a grapefruit knife, cut around the inside of the skin of grapefruit.
3. Cut out each segment, leaving behind all white pith.

Nut Butter Delight

Nut butters are delicious and healthy. Instead of peanut butter, try almond or cashew butter for a change of pace.

1/2 banana

1/2 cup (120 ml) whole milk

2 tablespoons (32 g) smooth almond or cashew butter

Combine the banana, milk, and nut butter in a blender; process until smooth. Add more milk, if needed.

YIELD: 1 toddler serving

EACH SERVING CONTAINS: 328.2 calories; 23.1 g total fat; 4.1 grams saturated fat; 12.2 mg cholesterol; 193.4 mg sodium; 25.8 g carbohydrates; 2.7 g dietary fiber; 9.4 g protein; 227.2 mg calcium; 1.4 mg iron; 162.5 IU vitamin A; and 5.4 mg vitamin C.

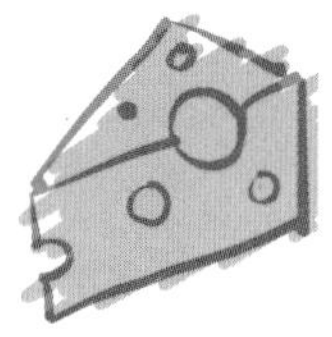

Eggs Florentine

Farmer's cheese or pot cheese is a soft, crumbly, unaged cheese that's similar to ricotta and queso blanco and high in protein.

2 eggs

1 tablespoon (15 g) full-fat cottage cheese

1 tablespoon (7 g) grated Swiss cheese

1 tablespoon (15 g) fresh farmer's cheese or pot cheese

½ teaspoon butter

¼ cup (40 g) thawed, drained, and chopped frozen spinach

Pinch grated nutmeg

OVEN METHOD: Preheat the oven to 350°F (180°C, gas mark 4). Grease a 6-ounce (175 ml) ramekin. Lightly beat the eggs in a small bowl, and add the cottage cheese, Swiss cheese, farmer's or pot cheese, and butter. Stir in the spinach and nutmeg. Pour the egg mixture into the prepared ramekin. Bake 30 minutes, or until a knife inserted in the center comes out clean. Remove and cool.

YIELD: 2 toddler servings, 3 tablespoons (45 g) each

EACH SERVING CONTAINS: 129.9 calories; 8.4 g total fat; 3.8 grams saturated fat; 227.7 mg cholesterol; 172.4 mg sodium; 2.9 g carbohydrates; 0.4 g dietary fiber; 9.2 g protein; 101.6 mg calcium; 1.0 mg iron; 1393.4 IU vitamin A; and 0.5 mg vitamin C.

Fabulously Fried Sweet Potatoes

Since toddlers have no real concept of breakfast, lunch, and dinner, it really doesn't matter what you serve when. The olive oil in this recipe helps the body absorb vitamin A from the sweet potato, and it might be well-received in the morning!

1 sweet potato

1 tablespoon (15 ml) olive oil

Scrub the sweet potato and prick its skin with a fork in several places. Microwave on high 5 minutes. Cool and peel the potato. Halve the potato lengthwise and cut each half into ½-inch (12 mm) slices.

Lightly coat a frying pan with oil and heat over medium heat. Add the potato slices, season lightly with salt if desired, and cook until nicely browned on the bottom. Turn the slices and cook 1 minute more until golden and crisp.

YIELD: 4 toddler servings, 2 slices each

EACH SERVING CONTAINS: 56.5 calories; 3.5 g total fat; 0.5 grams saturated fat; 0.0 mg cholesterol; 17.5 mg sodium; 5.8 g carbohydrates; 1.0 g dietary fiber; 0.5 g protein; 5.0 mg calcium; 0.2 mg iron; 1500.0 IU vitamin A; and 4.5 mg vitamin C.

Ga Ga Granola with Yogurt and Berries

This breakfast looks like dessert! What toddler wouldn't eat it up? Feel free to substitute different fruits based on what's in season and what your toddler enjoys most. Finely chopped almonds are also a healthy topping for this meal.

1/4 cup (30 g) Perfectly Plain Granola (page 158)

1/4 cup (60 g) plain yogurt

1/4 cup (36 g) mixed fresh blueberries and sliced strawberries

Pour the granola into a bowl and top with the yogurt and berries.

YIELD: 1 toddler serving

EACH SERVING CONTAINS: 116.2 calories; 12.9 g total fat; 3.0 grams saturated fat; 8.2 mg cholesterol; 30.5 mg sodium; 49.7 g carbohydrates; 6.6 g dietary fiber; 8.4 g protein; 107.3 mg calcium; 2.1 mg iron; 94.8 IU vitamin A; and 42.8 mg vitamin C.

I Want More Whole-Wheat Waffles ❄

For a treat, add fresh strawberries or peach slices and top with a little whipped cream.

3/4 cup (90 g) whole-wheat flour

3/4 cup (94 g) all-purpose flour

2 tablespoons (26 g) sugar

2 teaspoons baking powder

3/4 teaspoon baking soda

1/4 teaspoon salt

3 eggs (or 2 eggs plus 2 egg whites)

1 1/2 cups (355 ml) buttermilk

1/2 cup (112 g) butter, melted, or 1/2 cup (120 ml) olive oil

Preheat a waffle iron according to manufacturer's instructions. In a large bowl, combine the whole-wheat flour, all-purpose flour, sugar, baking powder, baking soda, and salt. Mix with a whisk or a fork. In a medium bowl, beat the eggs until blended and add the buttermilk and butter. Stir the wet ingredients into the dry ingredients. If the mixture seems too thick (it should pour off a spoon, not plop), add a bit of water.

Lightly oil the waffle iron. Pour the batter into the waffle iron and bake according to the manufacturer's instructions until crisp and golden. Repeat to make 6 waffles.

Leftover waffles, once cooled, may be frozen.

YIELD: 6 toddler servings, 1 waffle each

EACH SERVING (if using butter) CONTAINS: 315.3 calories; 17.9 g total fat; 11.8 grams saturated fat; 150.0 mg cholesterol; 683.6 mg sodium; 30.1 g carbohydrates; 2.3 g dietary fiber; 8.6 g protein; 219.1 mg calcium; 1.7 mg iron; 700.6 IU vitamin A; and 0.6 mg vitamin C.

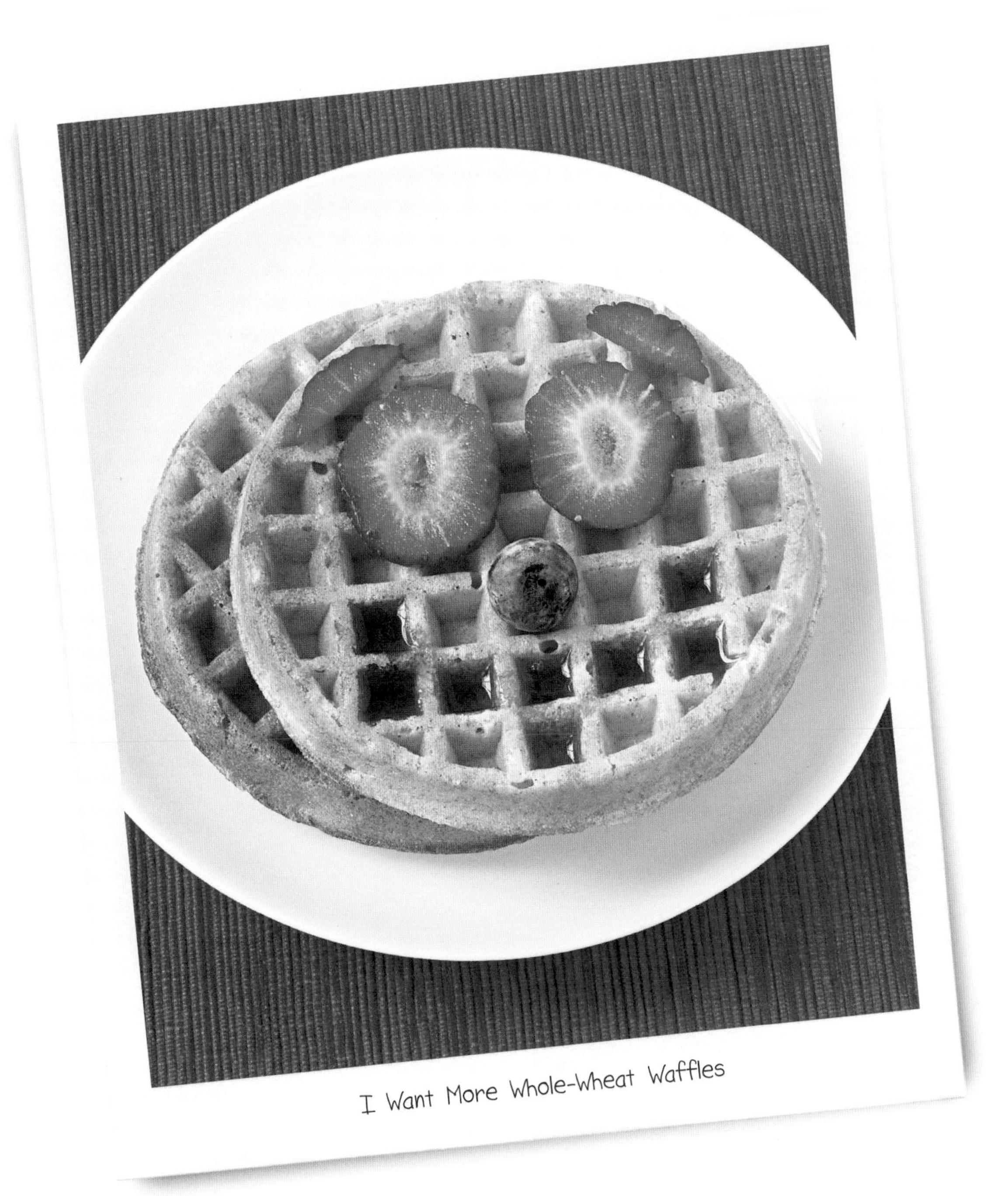

I Want More Whole-Wheat Waffles

Pleasing Pastina Breakfast

Pastina is an extremely small pasta shape made with durum wheat and egg. This recipe is extra delicious when served with fresh strawberries on the side.

¼ cup (44 g) cooked pastina

1 teaspoon butter

¼ cup (60 ml) whole fat milk

¼ mashed banana

MICROWAVE METHOD: Combine all ingredients in a microwave-safe bowl with lid. Microwave 20 seconds or until warm. Let stand 1 minute, then serve.

YIELD: 2 toddler servings, ¼ cup (55 g) each

EACH SERVING CONTAINS: 111.6 calories; 3.1 g total fat; 2.0 grams saturated fat; 8.1 mg cholesterol; 13.2 mg sodium; 18.4 g carbohydrates; 1.2 g dietary fiber; 3.2 g protein; 28.4 mg calcium; 0.5 mg iron; 116.4 IU vitamin A; and 2.5 mg vitamin C.

See How the Garden Grows

At twenty months, your toddler is still open to trying new foods. Continue to give him fresh fruits and vegetables when they're in season. A fun activity for the whole family is berry- or apple-picking, and most toddlers love to snack on fruit they've picked themselves. Combining fresh fruit with a protein such as cheese, milk, or peanut butter creates a well-balanced snack. Remember, your toddler still needs whole-milk dairy products, so don't switch to low-fat milk yet.

Date Sunrise Surprise

Dates have been enjoyed for centuries by people around the globe and are a good source of iron and potassium.

3 dates

½ cup (120 ml) orange juice

1 tablespoon (15 g) mashed banana

1 tablespoon (15 g) plain yogurt

1 tablespoon (15 g) Benjamin Bunny's Carrot Purée (page 154), or cooked and puréed leftover carrots

Pit and finely chop the dates. Combine with ¼ cup (60 ml) of the juice in a blender and process on high speed for 45 seconds until dates are well blended with the juice. Add the banana, yogurt, carrot purée, and remaining ¼ cup (60 ml) juice and blend well.

YIELD: 2 toddler servings, ⅓ cup (about 85 g) each

EACH SERVING CONTAINS: 73.8 calories; 0.7 g total fat; 0.3 grams saturated fat; 1.0 mg cholesterol; 39.1 mg sodium; 17.2 g carbohydrates; 1.6 g dietary fiber; 1.1 g protein; 18.6 mg calcium; 0.2 mg iron; 374.8 IU vitamin A; and 16.4 mg vitamin C.

Super Stuffed Tomatoes

Camparis are vine-ripened tomatoes, about 2 inches (5 cm) in diameter, with a wonderful flavor. If you can't find Campari tomatoes, use any vine-ripened variety.

2 Campari tomatoes

1 hard-cooked egg

1 teaspoon mayonnaise

1 small sprig fresh parsley

With a sharp knife, thinly slice off the bottom of each tomato. With a small spoon, scrape out the seeds and liquid of the tomatoes and discard. Cut the egg into small pieces. In a small bowl with a fork, mash the egg with the mayonnaise. Mince the parsley and stir into the egg. (You can omit the parsley from the egg filling and serve the sprig separately on the plate, next to the tomato, if you prefer.) With a small spoon, fill the tomatoes with the egg mixture. Cut in half and serve.

YIELD: 2 toddler servings, 1 tomato each

EACH SERVING CONTAINS: 54.9 calories; 4.1 g total fat; 1.0 grams saturated fat; 108.3 mg cholesterol; 52.5 mg sodium; 1.1 g carbohydrates; 0.2 g dietary fiber; 3.2 g protein; 14.5 mg calcium; 0.6 mg iron; 16.0 IU vitamin A; and 4.1 mg vitamin C.

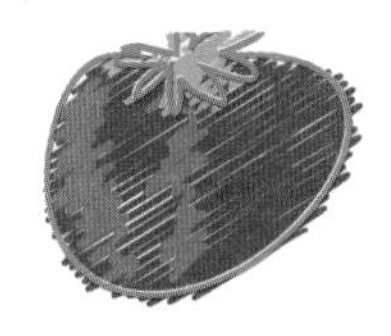

Yo-licious Topped Yogurt Cheese

This is as fun to eat as it is to make! See if your local grocer carries whole wheat waffle bowls to make it extra nutritious.

1 small ice-cream waffle bowl

¼ cup (60 g) yogurt cheese (page 104)

1 tablespoon (15 g) No Cook Prune Purée (page 47), Fuzzy Peach Purée (page 48), or mashed, fresh strawberries

Fill the ice-cream cone with the cheese and top with the prune or peach purée or strawberries.

YIELD: 1 toddler serving

EACH SERVING (if using fresh strawberries) CONTAINS: 97.7 calories; 1.2 g total fat; 0.1 grams saturated fat; 1.7 mg cholesterol; 68.2 mg sodium; 17.0 g carbohydrates; 0.3 g dietary fiber; 5.5 g protein; 115.2 mg calcium; 0.8 mg iron; 5.7 IU vitamin A; and 9.0 mg vitamin C.

Avocado in the Snow

Cut the egg halves in half again to make them easier for your toddler to handle.

1 hard-cooked egg

2 tablespoons (29 g) mashed avocado

Cut the egg in half and remove the yolk. Mash the avocado and yolk together. Spoon the mixture back into the hard-cooked egg halves.

YIELD: 2 toddler servings, ½ egg each

EACH SERVING CONTAINS: 59.0 calories; 4.5 g total fat; 1.1 grams saturated fat; 107.5 mg cholesterol; 33.6 mg sodium; 1.8 g carbohydrates; 1.0 g dietary fiber; 3.3 g protein; 11.8 mg calcium; 0.4 mg iron; 171.9 IU vitamin A; and 1.5 mg vitamin C.

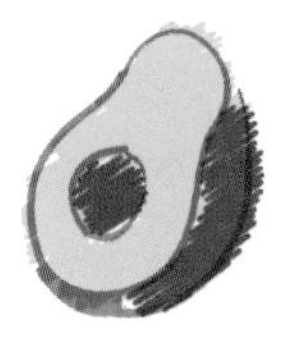

Emerald Nectar

This beverage can be made with or without the avocado. And don't be shy about finishing what your toddler doesn't. This is a healthy adult drink, too!

½ ripe avocado

1 cup (235 ml) apricot nectar

¼ cup (60 g) vanilla whole-milk yogurt

Peel and pit the avocado. Combine the avocado, apricot nectar, and yogurt in a blender and process until smooth.

YIELD: 4 toddler servings, ½ cup (120 ml) each

EACH SERVING CONTAINS: 84.7 calories; 4.2 g total fat; 0.9 grams saturated fat; 2.0 mg cholesterol; 10.7 mg sodium; 11.9 g carbohydrates; 2.1 g dietary fiber; 1.3 g protein; 26.0 mg calcium; 0.4 mg iron; 877.6 IU vitamin A; and 36.7 mg vitamin C.

Carrot-Peanut Butter Spread

This nutritious spread also works well with apple slices and celery sticks. It's also yummy for breakfast on finger-length slices of whole wheat toast.

½ cup (61 g) sliced carrots (about 3 small carrots)

2 tablespoons (28 ml) water

3 tablespoons (42 g) full-fat cottage cheese

1 tablespoon (18 g) frozen orange juice concentrate

2 teaspoons creamy peanut butter

Combine the carrots and water in a small microwave-safe bowl. Cover and microwave on high 3 minutes. Allow to cool slightly and then transfer to a blender. Add the cottage cheese, orange juice concentrate, and peanut butter and process 1 minute, or until the spread is smooth. If needed, use a spatula and scrape down the spread from the sides.

YIELD: 2 toddler servings, 2 heaping tablespoons (35 to 40 g) each

EACH SERVING CONTAINS: 81.0 calories; 3.4 g total fat; 1.2 grams saturated fat; 4.7 mg cholesterol; 129.6 mg sodium; 8.7 g carbohydrates; 1.2 g dietary fiber; 3.8 g protein; 25.6 mg calcium; 0.2 mg iron; 5383.4 IU vitamin A; and 11.6 mg vitamin C.

Radical Rice Cakes with Almond Butter

Avoid purchasing flavored rice cakes since many are high in sodium. Consider serving with ½ cup (120 ml) milk and ¼ cup (36 g) fresh blueberries.

2 mini rice cakes

2 teaspoons almond butter

Spread each rice cake with 1 teaspoon almond butter.

YIELD: 1 toddler serving

EACH SERVING CONTAINS: 102.4 calories; 6.6 g total fat; 0.7 grams saturated fat; 0.0 mg cholesterol; 61.9 mg sodium; 9.7 g carbohydrates; 0.6 g dietary fiber; 2.4 g protein; 30 mg calcium; 30.0 mg iron; 0.1 IU vitamin A; and 0.1 mg vitamin C.

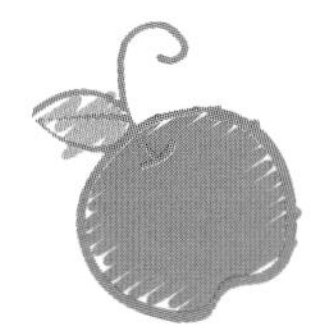

Avocado with Strawberry Cream Cheese

If your toddler is getting tired of the blandness of the avocado, try adding the fresh taste of strawberry cream cheese; it combines nicely with creamy avocado. The leftover filling is also good stuffed in fresh apricot halves or peaches or on top of pear or apple slices.

1 cup (230 g) cream cheese

½ cup (78 g) frozen or (80 g) dried pitted cherries

1 cup (170 g) sliced strawberries

1 avocado

Combine ½ cup (115 g) of the cream cheese and the cherries in a blender and process until smooth. Add the remaining ½ cup (115 g) of the cream cheese and the strawberries and continue processing until smooth. Peel, pit, and cut the avocado into quarters or eighths. Spread each avocado quarter or eighth with some of the strawberry cream cheese.

The strawberry cream cheese, tightly covered, will keep in the refrigerator for 2 to 3 days.

YIELD: Makes 24 (1-tablespoon) servings

EACH SERVING CONTAINS: 60.6 calories; 4.6 g total fat; 2.0 grams saturated fat; 10.7 mg cholesterol; 31.7 mg sodium; 5.8 g carbohydrates; 0.9 g dietary fiber; 0.9 g protein; 11.6 mg calcium; 0.8 mg iron; 362.8 IU vitamin A; and 5.0 mg vitamin C.

Banana-Raspberry Dream

The delicate raspberry is an excellent source of fiber. It's also high in antioxidants, B vitamins, and vitamin C.

1 small ripe banana

½ cup (65 g) fresh raspberries

½ cup (120 ml) whole vanilla soy milk

Place the banana, raspberries, and soy milk in a blender and process until smooth.

YIELD: 2 toddler servings, ½ cup (120 ml) each

EACH SERVING CONTAINS: 102.5 calories; 0.9 g total fat; 0.2 grams saturated fat; 0.0 mg cholesterol; 21.8 mg sodium; 23.7 g carbohydrates; 1.7 g dietary fiber; 2.6 g protein; 26.0 mg calcium; 0.5 mg iron; 37.8 IU vitamin A; and 11.1 mg vitamin C.

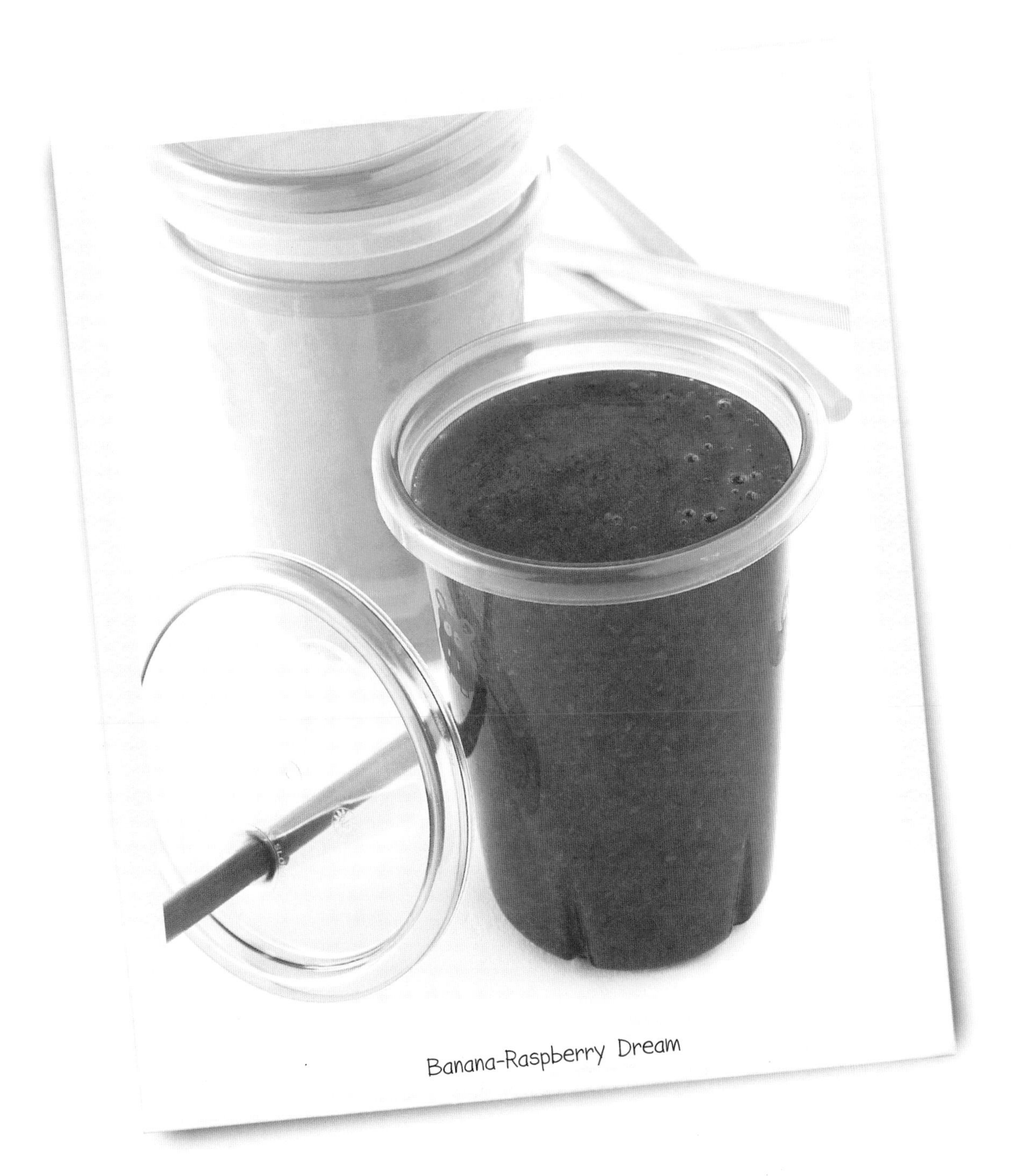

Banana-Raspberry Dream

Tuna Salad Surprise

This salad can be served with crackers, in pita bread with tomato, or as a sandwich. A toddler may prefer the tuna fish mixed only with mayonnaise. This makes a nice lunch served with pear slices and ½ cup (120 ml) whole milk.

1 can (6 ounces, or 170 g) water-packed chunk light tuna, drained

1 hard-cooked egg, chopped

2 tablespoons (28 g) mayonnaise

Combine the tuna, egg, and mayonnaise in a medium bowl. Mix well.

YIELD: 3 toddler servings, 2 heaping tablespoons (about 28 g) each

EACH SERVING CONTAINS: 152.5 calories; 9.6 g total fat; 1.5 grams saturated fat; 104.0 mg cholesterol; 330.7 mg sodium; 0.2 g carbohydrates; 0.0 g dietary fiber; 15.1 g protein; 8.3 mg calcium; 0.2 mg iron; 86.7 IU vitamin A; and 0.0 mg vitamin C.

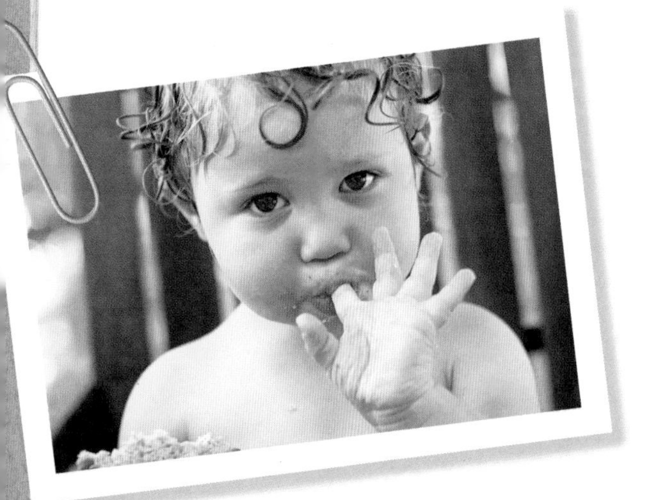

Stuffed Tomato with Tuna Salad Surprise

This recipe also works nicely with turkey or chicken salad.

1 small tomato

1 tablespoon (15 g) Tuna Salad Surprise (page 172)

Halve the tomato and scoop the seeds out. Stuff with the tuna salad.

YIELD: 1 toddler serving

EACH SERVING CONTAINS: 57.5 calories; 2.4 g total fat; 0.4 grams saturated fat; 3.8 mg cholesterol; 92.5 mg sodium; 6.1 g carbohydrates; 1.3 g dietary fiber; 2.5 g protein; 22.5 mg calcium; 0.8 mg iron; 1012.5 IU vitamin A; and 24.0 mg vitamin C.

Peanut Butter–Date Yummy Milk Shake

Smoothies are an excellent way for a child to get concentrated nutrients and calories in a small portion. Peanut butter and smooth nut butters are good sources of calories, zinc, and iron, which are important to a toddler's healthy growth and development.

4 soft pitted dates

1 tablespoon (16 g) smooth natural peanut butter

1/2 cup (120 ml) whole milk

Cut the dates into small pieces and combine with peanut butter and 1/4 cup (60 ml) of the milk in a blender. Process 30 to 45 seconds until completely smooth. Add the remaining milk and blend a few more seconds.

YIELD: 1 toddler serving, about 3/4 cup (175 ml)

EACH SERVING CONTAINS: 288.2 calories; 12.5 g total fat; 4.0 grams saturated fat; 12.2 mg cholesterol; 123.8 mg sodium; 41.0 g carbohydrates; 4.0 g dietary fiber; 8.4 g protein; 157.9 mg calcium; 0.6 mg iron; 124.4 IU vitamin A; and 0.0 mg vitamin C.

Very Berry Smoothie

Frozen mango works well in place of the mixed berries in this recipe, or feel free to experiment with what you have on hand!

1/2 cup (80 g) unsweetened mixed berries

1/2 banana

2 tablespoons (30 g) plain whole-milk yogurt

1 tablespoon (18 g) frozen orange juice concentrate

1 cup (235 ml) whole milk

Place the berries, banana, yogurt, orange juice concentrate, and milk in a blender and blend 60 seconds.

YIELD: 4 toddler servings, 1/2 cup (120 ml) each

EACH SERVING CONTAINS: 71.8 calories; 2.3 g total fat; 1.3 grams saturated fat; 7.1 mg cholesterol; 28.3 mg sodium; 10.9 g carbohydrates; 0.8 g dietary fiber; 2.6 g protein; 80.0 mg calcium; 0.1 mg iron; 89.2 IU vitamin A; and 8.0 mg vitamin C.

Very Veggie "Meat" Balls ❄

Serve these nutty vegetarian morsels plain with pasta and cheese or simmer them for a few minutes in tomato sauce and serve with spaghetti.

2 eggs

½ cup (50 g) pecans

⅓ cup (55 g) grated sweet onion

½ teaspoon salt (optional)

¾ cup (90 g) Italian-style seasoned bread crumbs

1 cup (120 g) grated 4-cheese Mexican blend or a mix of grated Cheddar and Monterey Jack cheese

1 teaspoon chopped fresh parsley

¼ cup (60 ml) olive oil

STOVETOP METHOD: In a blender, combine the eggs, pecans, onion, and salt (if using) and process until the nuts are completely ground. Transfer to a large bowl. Stir in the bread crumbs, mixing well. Mix in the cheese and parsley. Form 12 small balls. Heat the oil in a frying pan over medium heat. Add the balls and fry, turning often so they will not burn, for 10 minutes until nicely browned.

YIELD: 6 toddler servings, or 2 balls each

EACH SERVING CONTAINS: 277.1 calories; 20.8 g total fat; 4.6 grams saturated fat; 81.7 mg cholesterol; 395.3 mg sodium; 14.1 g carbohydrates; 2.1 g dietary fiber; 9.7 g protein; 104.6 mg calcium; 1.3 mg iron; 289.1 IU vitamin A; and 1.0 mg vitamin C.

Tasty Tuna Melt

Are you fishing for fast, convenient nutrition? This is a quick, tasty, open-faced sandwich. Serve with tomato slices and dill pickles.

1 tablespoon (14 g) mayonnaise

1 tablespoon (15 g) plain yogurt

1 can (5 ounces, or 140 g) chunk light tuna, packed in water, drained

1 slice whole-wheat bread

1 thin slice mozzarella cheese

OVEN METHOD: Preheat the broiler. Cover a baking sheet with tinfoil. In a medium bowl, combine the mayonnaise and yogurt; blend in the tuna. Spread half of the tuna evenly on the slice of bread and top it with the cheese. (Wrap and refrigerate the leftovers for your toddler's lunch tomorrow!) Place the open-faced sandwich on the prepared baking sheet. Broil until the cheese has melted. Let cool and cut the open-faced sandwich into bite-size pieces.

YIELD: 2 toddler servings, ½ sandwich each

EACH SERVING CONTAINS: 197.9 calories; 8.9 g total fat; 2.3 grams saturated fat; 46.0 mg cholesterol; 503.9 mg sodium; 7.3 g carbohydrates; 1.2 g dietary fiber; 21.1 g protein; 100.5 mg calcium; 0.4 mg iron; 108.1 IU vitamin A; and 0.0 mg vitamin C.

Popeye's Favorite Spinach Salad

Serve this with soup, a sandwich, and melon for dessert. Note that your toddler may prefer to eat the salad as finger food, without the dressing.

1/4 small bunch spinach (about 3/4 cup, or 25 g)

1 small slice cooked bacon

1/2 hard-cooked egg

2 small white mushrooms

Wonderfully Warm Sherry Vinaigrette, optional (see right)

Wash, dry, and remove the stems from the spinach. Tear into pieces and place in a salad bowl. Tear the bacon into pieces and add to the spinach. Chop the egg and slice the mushrooms and add to mixture. Add the dressing (if using) and toss gently.

YIELD: 1 toddler serving

EACH SERVING (not including optional vinaigrette) CONTAINS: 67.5 calories; 68.1 g total fat; 1.5 grams saturated fat; 112.5 mg cholesterol; 120.9 mg sodium; 1.8 g carbohydrates; 0.6 g dietary fiber; 5.4 g protein; 34.2 mg calcium; 1.0 mg iron; 2259.8 IU vitamin A; and 6.3 mg vitamin C.

Wonderfully Warm Sherry Vinaigrette

This lovely dressing is great with any green salad, either for you or for your little one.

6 tablespoons (90 ml) olive oil

3 tablespoons (45 ml) sherry vinegar

1/2 teaspoon Dijon mustard

1/4 teaspoon salt

Pinch freshly ground pepper

MICROWAVE METHOD: In a small, lidded microwave-safe container, combine the oil, vinegar, mustard, salt, and pepper; shake until you have a creamy consistency. Remove the lid and warm in the microwave on high 30 seconds.

YIELD: 8 toddler servings, 1 tablespoon (15 ml) each

EACH SERVING CONTAINS: 94.8 calories; 10.5 g total fat; 1.5 grams saturated fat; 0.0 mg cholesterol; 80.2 mg sodium; 0.1 g carbohydrates; 0.0 g dietary fiber; 0.0 g protein; 0.0 mg calcium; 0.0 mg iron; 0.0 IU vitamin A; and 0.0 mg vitamin C.

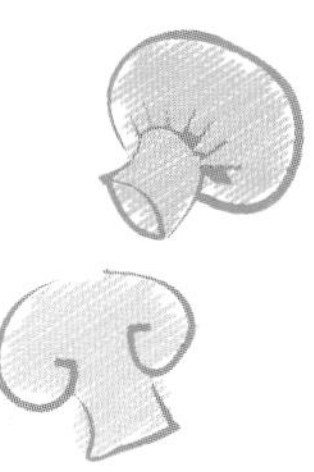

Cucumber, Shrimp, and Spinach Salad

Your toddler may prefer this salad plain or lightly drizzled with dressing. If you don't have shrimp, use leftover cooked chicken.

1 cup (30 g) packed fresh spinach leaves, washed

4 slices peeled cucumber

2 or 3 large cooked shrimp

Creamy Lemon Dressing (see right)

STOVETOP METHOD: With water droplets still clinging to the leaves, cook the spinach in a small skillet over medium heat for 2 minutes, tossing, until soft. Drain the spinach, let cool, and squeeze into a square shape. Place the cucumbers on a plate in a nice pattern. Peel the shrimp and remove the tails. Cut into small pieces and arrange on top of the cucumbers. Place the spinach next to the cucumbers. Drizzle with Creamy Lemon Dressing (optional).

YIELD: 1 toddler serving

EACH SERVING (not including Creamy Lemon Dressing) CONTAINS: 50.0 calories; 0.5 g total fat; 0.0 grams saturated fat; 57.4 mg cholesterol; 128.7 mg sodium; 3.9 g carbohydrates; 1.8 g dietary fiber; 8.2 g protein; 49.0 mg calcium; 1.7 mg iron; 1202.1 IU vitamin A; and 7.3 mg vitamin C.

Creamy Lemon Dressing

This is a great all-around dressing for any salad. To make it family-size, use 1 cup (230 g) yogurt, 4 teaspoons (20 ml) vinegar and 2 teaspoons lemon juice.

2 tablespoons (20 g) plain whole-milk yogurt

½ teaspoon white wine vinegar

¼ teaspoon lemon juice

Combine the yogurt, vinegar, and lemon juice and whisk together vigorously with a fork.

YIELD: 1 toddler serving

EACH SERVING CONTAINS: 19.6 calories; 1.0 g total fat; 0.6 grams saturated fat; 4.0 mg cholesterol; 14.1 mg sodium; 1.8 g carbohydrates; 0.0 g dietary fiber; 1.1 g protein; 37.3 mg calcium; 0.0 mg iron; 31.1 IU vitamin A; and 1.9 mg vitamin C.

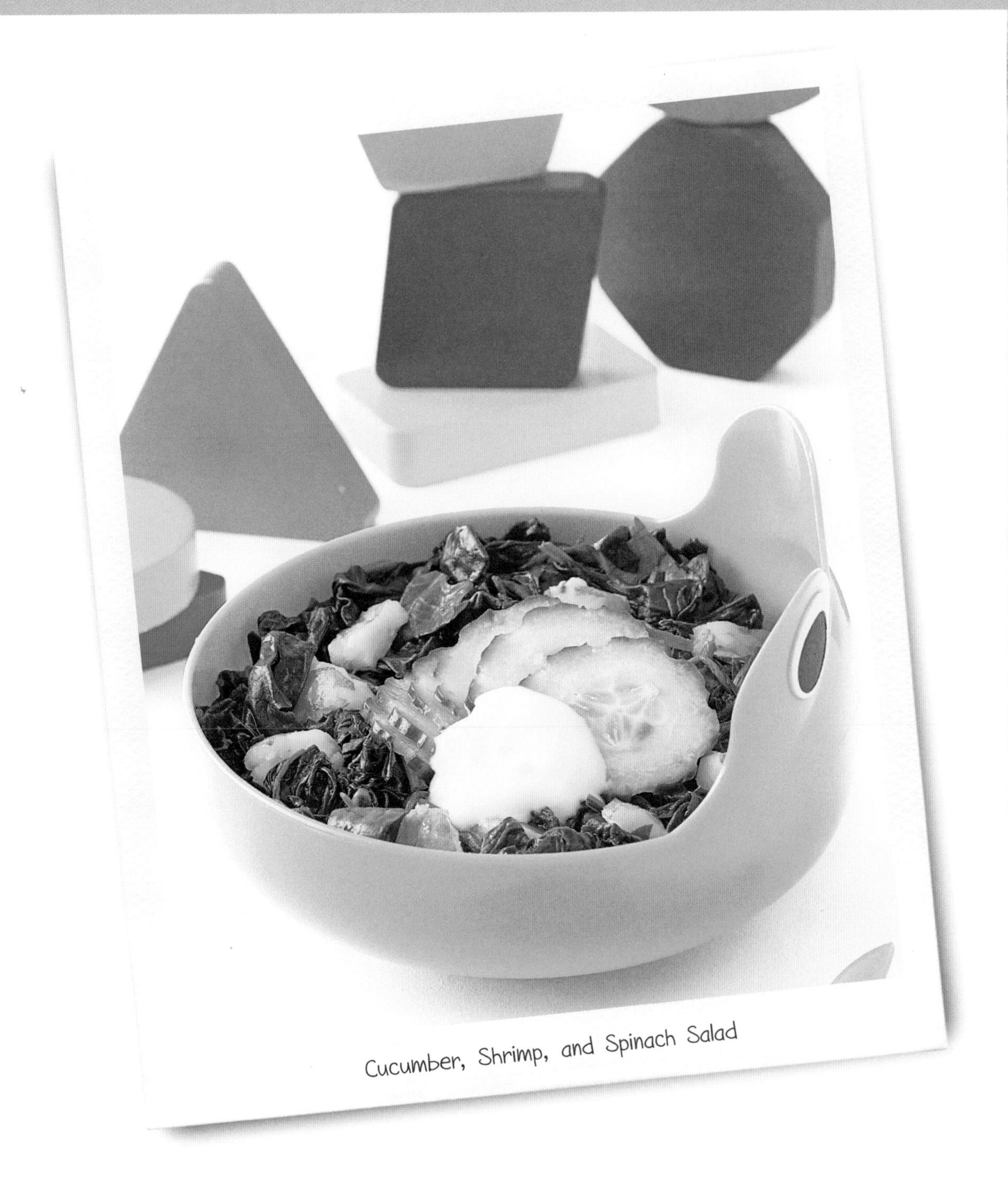

Cucumber, Shrimp, and Spinach Salad

Make It a Meal: The Amazing Artichoke

Artichokes are available year-round, but their peak season is spring. It's then they are least expensive. Look for ones that are bright green and have leaves that are tightly packed and blemish free.

HOW TO PREPARE

Before cooking artichokes, do the following:

1. Wash them.
2. Pull off outer lower leaves toward the base and discard.
3. Cut off the stem and discard.
4. With a pair of scissors, snip thorny tips off the remaining petals and cut off the top quarter of the artichoke. Discard.

HOW TO COOK

Cooking artichokes is really simple. Just follow these easy steps:

STOVETOP METHOD: Steam 40 to 45 minutes until a leaf comes out easily. Or, stand up in a pan with 3 inches (7.5 cm) of water. Cover and boil gently 25 to 45 minutes, according to size. Stand upside down to drain.

MICROWAVE METHOD: Invert 1 large prepared artichoke in a deep 1-quart (946 ml) microwave-safe cup or bowl. Add 1/3 cup (75 ml) water. Cover and microwave on high 7 minutes. Let stand 5 minutes. When done, petals will pull out easily.

HOW TO EAT

Your toddler may enjoy the ritual of eating an artichoke. To eat, pull off petals one at the time. Dunk base of petal into melted butter; pull the very bottom of the leaf through teeth to scrape off the soft, pulpy portion of the petal. When all the petals have been removed, spoon out and discard the fuzzy stuff (the choke) at the base. The bottom, or heart, is completely edible and incredibly delicious.

Yummy Recipe Tip: Artichoke Dips

Here are a number of different dips that work well with artichokes:

- 1/4 cup (60 g) mayonnaise and 1/2 teaspoon lemon juice
- 1/4 cup (60 g) mayonnaise and 1 teaspoon pesto
- 2 tablespoons (28 g) mayonnaise, 2 tablespoons (30 g) sour cream or plain yogurt, and 1/2 teaspoon lemon juice
- 1 tablespoon (15 g) mayonnaise, 1 tablespoon (15 g) sour cream, 1/4 teaspoon mustard, 1/2 teaspoon ketchup, and 1 tablespoon (15 ml) fresh orange juice.

Yes, Yes, Yogurt Sauce and Eggplant

Eggplant is best between August and October. It's an important source of fiber, vitamins, minerals, and antioxidants. Serve the eggplant with cooked basmati rice. The flavor combination is really nice.

1 tablespoon (15 ml) olive oil

1 small eggplant (about 1 pound, or 455 g)

Dash of salt

½ cup (115 g) plain yogurt

STOVETOP METHOD: Lightly coat a frying pan with some of the olive oil and heat over medium heat. Cut eggplant into ½-inch (12 mm) slices. Sprinkle each slice lightly with salt and brush both sides with olive oil. Place the eggplant in the frying pan. Cook 10 minutes until the eggplant is browned. Turn and cook the other side until browned. Allow to cool and then remove skin from the eggplant. Warm the yogurt over low heat and pour over the eggplant.

YIELD: 8 toddler servings, or 1 slice each

EACH SERVING CONTAINS: 38.7 calories; 2.4 g total fat; 0.6 grams saturated fat; 2.0 mg cholesterol; 8.2 mg sodium; 4.0 g carbohydrates; 1.9 g dietary fiber; 1.1 g protein; 23.7 mg calcium; 0.1 mg iron; 30.5 IU vitamin A; and 1.3 mg vitamin C.

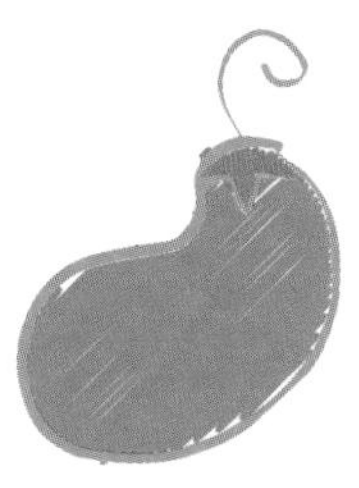

Broccoli-Cheddar Soup

Serve this soup with whole-wheat bread and slices of a ripe pear washed and cored.

2 tablespoons (28 ml) olive oil

1 small onion

1 leek, white part only

1 teaspoon chopped garlic

2 small potatoes

1 pound (455 g) broccoli

2 cans (14 ounces, or 425 ml each) vegetable or nonfat chicken broth or 3 cups (700 ml) homemade broth

1½ cups (355 ml) whole milk

½ to 1 cup (60 to 120 g) packed, grated Cheddar cheese

STOVETOP METHOD: Heat the oil in a large saucepan over low heat. Peel and chop the onion and sauté 5 minutes. Clean and slice the leak, and add leak and garlic to saucepan and continue to sauté 5 more minutes, stirring occasionally. Wash, peel, and cube the potatoes. Wash and chop the broccol. Add both as well as the broth to the saucepan. Cover and simmer 30 minutes or until the vegetables are soft. Allow to cool slightly and then pulse or purée the mixture (depending on how smooth you like your soup) in two batches in the blender. Add some of the milk if you need to thin the soup. Return the soup to the pan, add the milk, and gently reheat. Stir in the cheese until melted.

YIELD: Makes 6 toddler servings, 1 cup (235 ml) each

EACH SERVING CONTAINS: 155.1 calories; 5.9 g total fat; 1.4 grams saturated fat; 8.1 mg cholesterol; 450.4 mg sodium; 15.4 g carbohydrates; 3.1 g dietary fiber; 7.6 g protein; 65.5 mg calcium; 0.4 mg iron; 199.0 IU vitamin A; and 31.4 mg vitamin C.

Perfect Petite Pesto

This is a small-portion recipe for pesto. You may want to double or triple it. It freezes well and is a favorite on spaghetti. If you can't find pine nuts, walnuts will work.

½ cup (20 g) firmly packed fresh basil

1 teaspoon minced, fresh garlic

1 tablespoon (9 g) pine nuts

3 tablespoons (45 ml) extra virgin olive oil

1 tablespoon (5 g) firmly packed grated Parmesan or Romano

Salt and pepper (optional)

Wash and dry basil and place in a blender with garlic and pine nuts. Pulse into a coarse paste. Slowly add olive oil and process until all the ingredients are well blended. Transfer mixture to a bowl using a spatula. Stir in the cheese and season with salt and pepper, if desired.

YIELD: 4 toddler servings, or 2 tablespoons (15 g) each

EACH SERVING CONTAINS: 131.9 calories; 13.5 g total fat; 2.4 grams saturated fat; 1.9 mg cholesterol; 33.9 mg sodium; 0.9 g carbohydrates; 0.4 g dietary fiber; 1.5 g protein; 32.6 mg calcium; 0.4 mg iron; 279.8 IU vitamin A; and 1.0 mg vitamin C.

Starry Night Broccoli Pasta

Using little pasta shapes make this an appealing meal for toddlers. If you can't find stelline, use alphabet pasta, farfalle (bowties), or rotelle (wheels). For the tubular pasta, ditalini or small elbows are both good choices.

2 tablespoons (22 g) uncooked stelline (star-shaped) pasta

1 tablespoon (7 g) uncooked short, tubular pasta

3 or 4 small broccoli pieces

Grated Parmesan or Romano, to taste

STOVETOP METHOD: Bring 1 cup (235 ml) water to a boil in a medium saucepan. Add the both pastas, and reduce heat; simmer 5 minutes. Add the broccoli and cook 5 minutes more, stirring occasionally, until the pasta is soft and the broccoli is cooked. Add a little more water if the pasta becomes too dry. At the end of cooking, the water should be mostly absorbed by the pasta. Transfer the pasta and broccoli to a plate or bowl. Sprinkle with the cheese and let cool slightly before serving to your toddler.

YIELD: 1 toddler serving, or ½ cup (115 g)

EACH SERVING CONTAINS: 121.7 calories; 0.7 g total fat; 0.2 grams saturated fat; 0.0 mg cholesterol; 20.3 mg sodium; 24.0 g carbohydrates; 2.4 g dietary fiber; 5.9 g protein; 67.0 mg calcium; 2.2 mg iron; 1495.8 IU vitamin A; and 11.5 mg vitamin C.

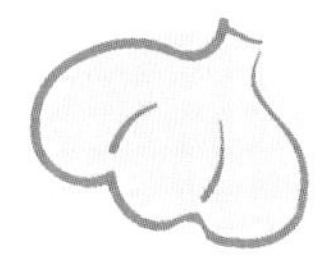

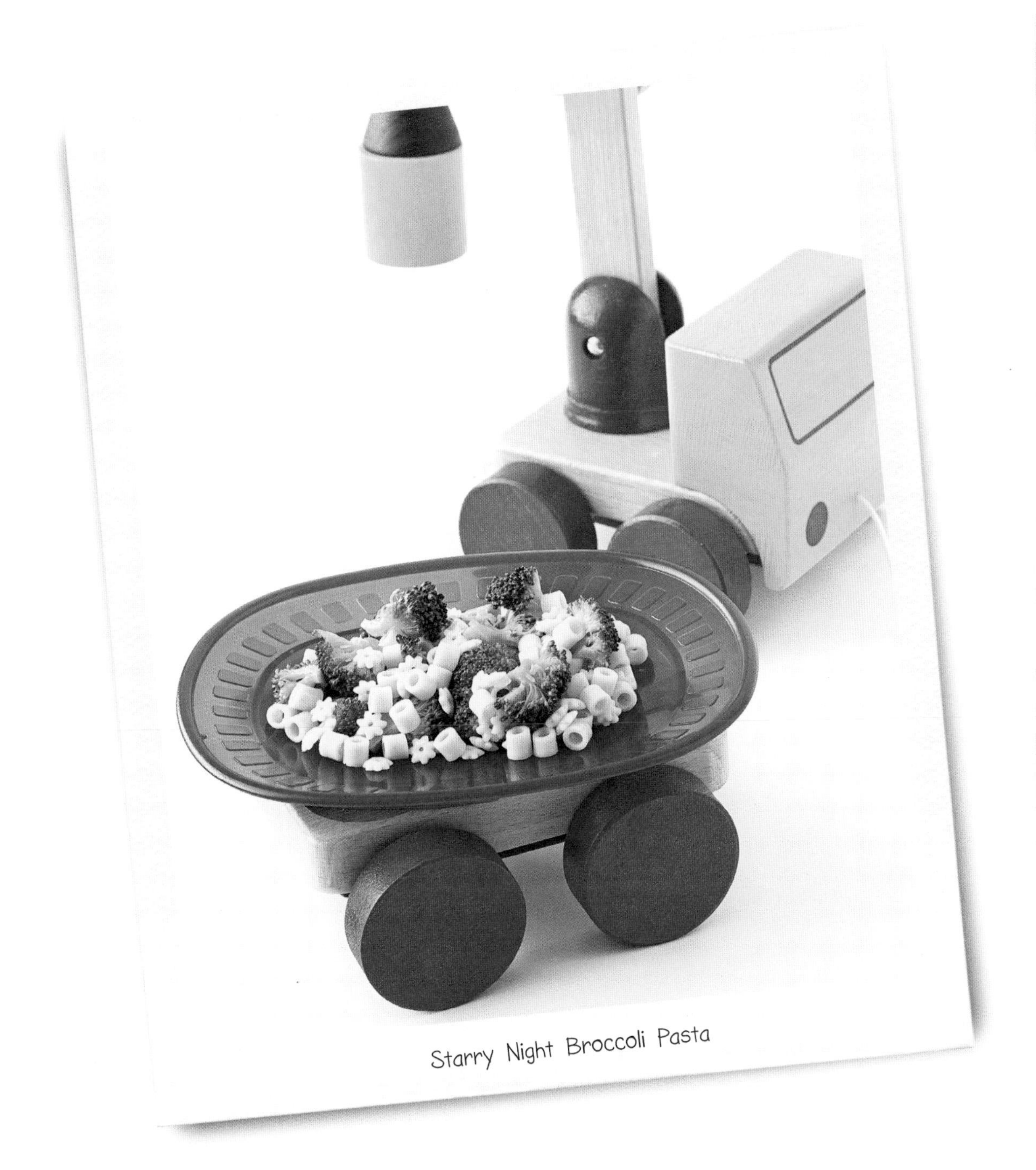

Starry Night Broccoli Pasta

Rice, Veggie, Fruit Medley

If you have leftover vegetables, this is a quick and simple dinner for a hungry and impatient toddler. If you need to cook the rice, use quick-cooking instant rice.

2 tablespoons (21 g) cooked rice

1 tablespoon (15 g) chopped carrots, green beans, corn, zucchini, asparagus, or peas

1 tablespoon (11 g) chopped tomato or (9 g) avocado

1 tablespoon (10 g) chopped melon, peach, pear, or orange

Reheat the rice. Microwave or steam the vegetables of choice. Mix together the rice, vegetables, tomato or avocado, and fruit of choice.

YIELD: 1 toddler serving

EACH SERVING (if using melon) CONTAINS: 36.4 calories; 0.1 g total fat; 0.0 grams saturated fat; 0.0 mg cholesterol; 32.6 mg sodium; 8.0 g carbohydrates; 0.5 g dietary fiber; 0.8 g protein; 13.6 mg calcium; 0.4 mg iron; 1734.6 IU vitamin A; and 5.9 mg vitamin C.

Tiny Tasty Chicken Nuggets ❄

These are tasty and quick to make—and much healthier than fast-food chicken nuggets. For the coating, grind bread crumbs seasoned with a little salt, pepper, and oregano in the blender or use tempura or panko crumbs.

1 tablespoon (15 ml) olive oil, or more as needed

1 egg

1 tablespoon (15 ml) whole milk

1/4 cup (30 g) seasoned bread crumbs

3 boneless and skinless chicken breasts, cut into nugget-size pieces

OVEN AND STOVETOP METHOD: Preheat the oven to 400°F (200°C, gas mark 6). Heat the oil in a frying pan over medium-high heat. Whisk the egg and milk in a bowl. Place the bread crumbs on a plate. Dip each piece of chicken first in the egg/milk mixture and then dredge in the bread crumbs, covering both sides. Cook in the hot oil 1 minute; turn and cook 1 minute more. Place the chicken in a baking dish and bake 15 minutes or until meat is cooked through and any juices run clear. (Meat thermometer should register 160 to 180°F [71 to 82°C].)

YIELD: 12 toddler servings, 4 nuggets each

EACH SERVING CONTAINS: 175.3 calories; 12.2 g total fat; 2.5 grams saturated fat; 72.5 mg cholesterol; 217.9 mg sodium; 7.8 g carbohydrates; 0.6 g dietary fiber; 8.3 g protein; 13.3 mg calcium; 0.7 mg iron; 75.0 IU vitamin A; and 0.0 mg vitamin C.

Avocado, Cucumber, and Tomato Salad

Technically, a cucumber is a fruit, but it's grouped into the veggie family due to its uses. Your toddler will love the cucumber's clean taste but may prefer the salad without dressing.

½ avocado

¼ cucumber

½ large, ripe tomato

Dressing of choice (optional)

Peel, pit, and cube the avocado. Peel and slice the cucumber and then halve the slices. Wash and cube the tomato. Combine the avocado, cucumber, and tomato into a bowl and toss lightly with the dressing.

YIELD: 2 toddler servings, ⅓ cup (about 85 g) each

EACH SERVING (not including optional dressing) CONTAINS: 90.4 calories; 7.4 g total fat; 1.1 grams saturated fat; 0.0 mg cholesterol; 8.5 mg sodium; 6.3 g carbohydrates; 4.0 g dietary fiber; 1.6 g protein; 18.6 mg calcium; 0.6 mg iron; 399.1 IU vitamin A; and 13.3 mg vitamin C.

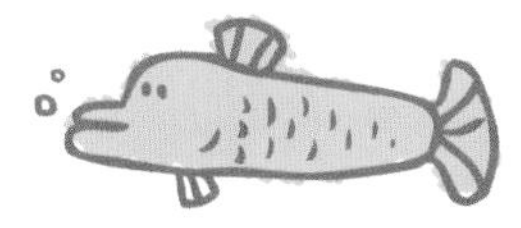

Happy Haddock and Tomatoes

Haddock is a mild white fish high in vitamin B12 and protein and similar in taste to cod. This quick, easy, and mouth-watering recipe goes well with mashed potatoes and green beans.

2 tablespoons (28 g) butter

4 ounces (115 g) frozen haddock, without skin and bone, partially defrosted

Juice of lemon wedge

Salt (optional)

¼ tomato, cut in two

2 teaspoons fresh chopped parsley

STOVETOP METHOD: Melt the butter in a heavy-bottomed pan over medium-low heat. Cut the fish into two pieces. Add the fish to the pan and sprinkle with the lemon juice and a little salt (if using). Place the two tomato wedges around the fish. Cover the pan and simmer 5 to 10 minutes until the fish flakes easily when prodded with a fork. Do not overcook the fish or it will be dry. Sprinkle with the parsley.

YIELD: 2 toddler servings, 2 ounces (55 g) each

EACH SERVING CONTAINS: 206.3 calories; 15.9 g total fat; 9.1 grams saturated fat; 45.6 mg cholesterol; 204.1 mg sodium; 8.7 g carbohydrates; 1.1 g dietary fiber; 7.3 g protein; 13.2 mg calcium; 0.5 mg iron; 631.7 IU vitamin A; and 4.7 mg vitamin C.

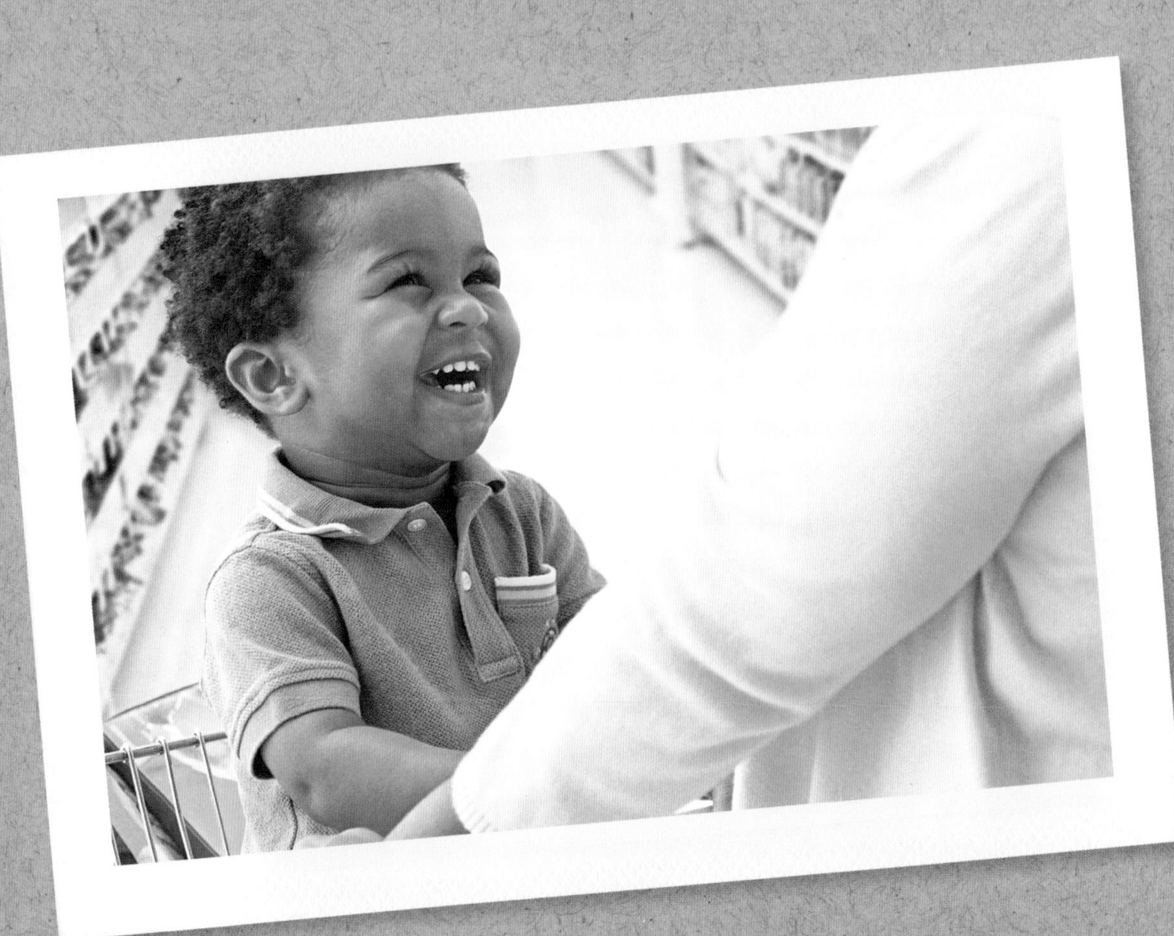

"There are two lasting bequests we can give our children.
One is roots. The other is wings."
— Hodding Carter, Jr.

CHAPTER FOUR

Getting the Best Early Nutrition—A Reference for Your Baby and Toddler

Good nutrition is important to our health and well being. Understanding the basic elements that constitute good nutrition is helpful when you want to foster healthy eating habits among your family.

Use the following chapter as a reference guide to understanding nutrition and the role good nutrition plays in your child's life. Remember, it's up to you to set the proper foundation for a lifetime of healthy eating.

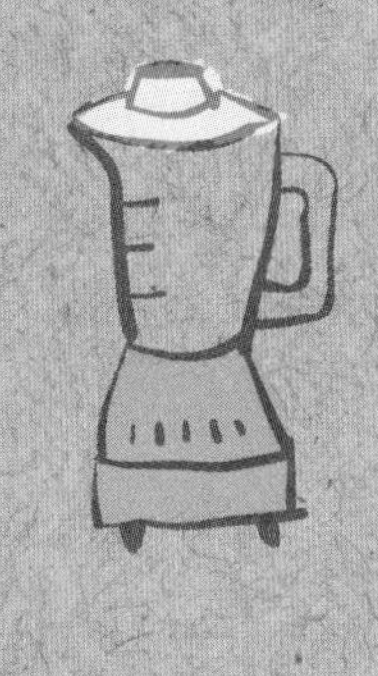

All About: Protein

WHAT IT DOES: Protein is important for growth, energy, and tissue repair. The brain, muscles, blood, skin, hair, nails, and connective tissues are predominantly made of protein. Protein also transports hormones and vitamins through the bloodstream, builds muscle, forms antibodies for the immune system, and plays an essential role in maintaining the body's fluid balance.

SOURCES: Primary sources of protein include red meat, pork, poultry, fish, milk, yogurt, cheese, and eggs. (Animal sources of protein are sometimes called "complete" protein because they provide all twenty-two essential amino acids that the body needs.) Soy, though from a plant, provides the best source of non-animal protein. Secondary sources of protein (or "incomplete" protein) include beans, lentils, rice, bread, cereals, vegetables, grains, nuts, and seeds.

HOW MUCH DOES MY CHILD NEED?: Up to six months of age, most babies receive all the protein they need from breast milk or formula. Between six and twelve months of age, food supplements an infant's protein requirements. Toddlers (one to two years) need about 16 grams of protein each day. Two cups (475 ml) of whole milk each day plus 1 ounce (28 g) of beef, poultry, or fish should be enough to meet their requirements.

All About: Carbohydrates

WHAT THEY DO: Carbohydrates are our bodies' main energy source.

SOURCES: There are two kinds of carbohydrates: simple and complex. Simple carbohydrates are made up of simple sugars such as table sugar (sucrose), honey, corn syrup, and molasses. They provide quick energy, but they have little nutritional value and are often categorized as "empty calories." However, these sugars are also present in fruit, vegetables, and milk, which add necessary vitamins, minerals, and fiber to the diet.

Complex carbohydrates contribute starch and fiber to the diet and may also supply protein and important vitamins and minerals. Complex carbohydrates are absorbed more slowly than simple carbohydrates, giving the body a more continuous source of energy.

Complex carbohydrates come from grains, beans and legumes, and vegetables:

- **Breads:** Whole-grain breads are good sources of complex carbohydrates. Multigrain, buckwheat, whole-wheat, barley, rye, and oat breads are excellent choices. When made with enriched white flour, crackers, pizza dough, buns, tortillas, and other flat breads are also sources of carbohydrates, but they're not as nutritious as their whole-grain cousins, so give them to your child only on occasion.
- **Cereals, Pasta, and Rice:** Whole-grain wheat, rye, oat, and barley cereals— hot or cold—are good sources of carbohydrates, along with pasta, polenta (cornmeal), rice (brown), couscous (made from semolina flour), and kasha (buckwheat).
- **Beans, Legumes, and Veggies:** Dried beans, lentils, and peanuts are all good sources of complex carbohydrates, as are potatoes, sweet potatoes, yams, corn, and squash.

HOW MUCH DOES MY CHILD NEED?: There is no Reference Daily Intake (RDI) for carbohydrates, but a balanced diet will provide an adequate supply for babies. For toddlers, 50 to 60 percent of their calories should come from nutrient-rich carbohydrates, and foods with added sugar (such as candy and soda) should be served only on special occasions.

Why Choose Whole Grains?

Health and nutrition experts always recommend that you choose products made with whole grains. That's because they have vitamins and minerals that refined grains don't. While refined products may be fortified, this doesn't make up for all the important nutrients and fiber that were removed. When buying bread, bread products, and cereals, look for whole wheat flour, rolled oats, whole grain, or stone-ground whole grains as the first ingredient.

All About: Dietary Fiber

WHAT IT DOES: Fiber aids digestion, lowers cholesterol levels, and may reduce the risk of heart disease and obesity later in life. Fiber also helps prevent constipation, a frequent problem for many children.

TYPES: Dietary fiber, which is found only in plants, is divided into two categories: soluble and insoluble.

- **Soluble fiber** dissolves within the digestive system and generally passes through the body without being absorbed. It expands and becomes gel-like on contact with water. Soluble fiber can help lower cholesterol levels.
- **Insoluble fiber,** or roughage, passes through the intestines virtually unchanged. Insoluble fiber adds bulk to the stool and speeds transit time through the intestines, potentially reducing the risk of colon cancer.

SOURCES: Soluble fiber is found in peanuts, lentils, beans, barley, oats, and oat bran. Other excellent sources of soluble fiber are fresh fruits and vegetables, especially blackberries, unpeeled apples and pears, avocados, peas, artichokes, parsnips, prunes, and dried dates. Insoluble fiber is found in all whole grains, wheat bran, fruit and vegetable skins, corn kernels, and seeds.

Butter vs. Margarine: What Is Best for Your Baby?

Butter and margarine are major sources of dietary fat. Butter has 100 calories, 30 milligrams of cholesterol, and 7 grams of saturated fat per tablespoon (15 g). Margarine has between 45 and 100 calories, 0 milligrams of cholesterol, and 1 to 2 grams of saturated fat per tablespoon (15 g). While supermarkets now carry margarine without trans fat, we like using butter for baby. It's pure and natural. Most margarines contain highly processed vegetable oils, soy protein isolate, and an assortment of additives.

HOW MUCH DOES MY CHILD NEED?: For infants under two years of age, there is no recommendation for total fiber. A balanced diet with plenty of whole grains, vegetables, and fruits will easily provide all the fiber your baby needs. For children three years of age, experts recommend 5 grams of fiber plus the child's age, so a three-year-old would need 8 grams of fiber per day, a four year old would need 9 grams per day, and a five year old 10 grams per day.

Keep in mind that you don't need to calculate your child's fiber intake in grams. A minimum of three daily servings of green and/or yellow vegetables, two servings of fruit, and four to six servings of whole-grain bread, crackers, pasta, or cereal will provide an adequate amount of fiber. It's important to remember that those grain servings should be whole grains, which always have more fiber than products made with white flour. On ingredient labels, look for the words "whole wheat" or "whole grain." (Wheat flour does not mean it contains whole wheat.)

In some cases, there can be such a thing as too much fiber. A diet rich in whole grains, vegetables, and fruit provides all the fiber a toddler needs. Some well-meaning parents may feed their babies a diet high in fiber and low in fat. This is not recommended for infants and toddlers under two years old.

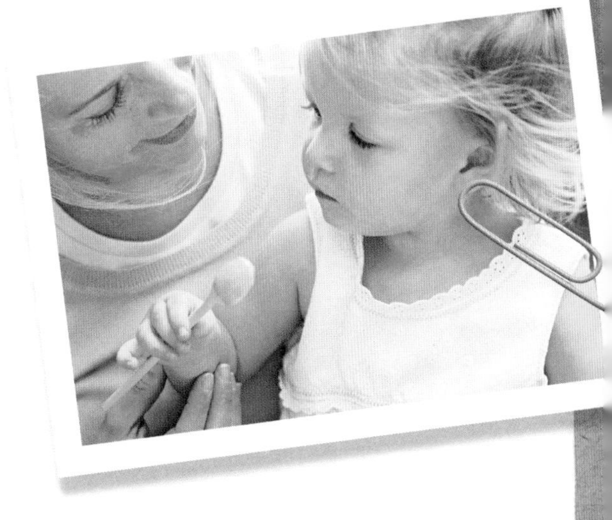

All About: Fat

WHAT IT DOES: Fat is probably one of the most misunderstood nutrients in food. In fact, fat is important to good health and also helps regulate our eating habits. Having nine calories per gram, fat is the best supplier of energy. This is especially important when it comes to baby and toddler diets. Fat insulates against temperature changes, provides a protective cushion for vital organs, and keeps skin and hair healthy. Fat also helps the body absorb the four fat-soluble vitamins: A, D, E, and K. Because fat is digested and absorbed slowly, delaying gastric emptying, meals eaten with fat cause greater satiety and turn off the desire to eat too much or too often.

TYPES: It's important to note that not all fats are created equal; some are much better for you than others. Even so, there should not be any restrictions of fats among infants and toddlers—except for trans fats, which should be avoided. The calories from fat are necessary during these crucial growing years, and fat also plays an important role in brain development. There are three types of fat in addition to trans fats:

- **Polyunsaturated fats** lower total blood cholesterol, but they also lower HDL (the "good" cholesterol).
- **Monounsaturated fats** may help lower blood cholesterol, thereby reducing risk of cardiovascular disease.
- **Saturated fat** is needed in babies' and toddlers' diets to support growth and development.
- **Trans fats** are considered harmful because they tend to act like saturated fat and raise LDL ("bad") cholesterol and lower HDL ("good") cholesterol. Trans fats are created when polyunsaturated vegetable oils are hydrogenated to create a spreadable fat that's solid at room temperature.

What Are the Best Types of Vegetable Oil?

Olive oil is a healthy alternative to margarine and butter; it contains no cholesterol, very little saturated fat, and mostly monounsaturated fat. Other mostly polyunsaturated vegetable oils that contain no cholesterol are corn, cottonseed, peanut, soy bean, safflower, and sunflower oils.

Are you confused about all the different olive oils available? Extra-virgin, virgin, regular, or light olive oils all have the same amount of calories per tablespoon. The descriptions refer to the taste or processing of the oil, not to the amount of fat or calories. The olive oils are graded in accordance with the degree of acidity they contain. (Extra-virgin has the lowest acidity, with about 1 percent.)

SOURCES: Breast milk and whole milk are good sources of fat calories since infants and toddlers cannot eat meat, nuts, butter, or oil in adequate quantities to supply enough calories. (Too much saturated fat in an adult's diet may raise cholesterol levels, increasing the risk for heart disease.)

Fat exists in both plants and animals. It is abundant in meats, dairy products, butter, shortening, salad and cooking oils, poultry, fish, and fatty vegetables such as avocados, soy beans, and olives. All fats in food are combinations of saturated, monounsaturated, and polyunsaturated fats. However, certain foods are higher in one type of fat than in others:

- Good sources of polyunsaturated fats include sunflower, corn, soy bean, cottonseed, and safflower oils.
- Monounsaturated fats are abundant in olive oil, canola oil, pecans, cashews, macadamia nuts, peanuts, pistachio nuts, and avocados.
- Saturated fats are found in large amounts in red meat, pork, cream, whole milk and whole milk dairy products, coconut milk, coconut oil, cocoa butter, and palm kernel oils.
- Trans fats are found in most vegetable shortenings, occasionally in margarine, and also in many snack foods such as crackers, cookies, cakes, pastries, and chips, as well as in fried foods and processed convenience foods such as frozen pizza, boxed macaroni and cheese, and toaster pastries. The amount of trans fat is now listed on the nutrition label of all foods. Look for zero trans fats on the nutrition label and the absence of partially hydrogenated oils in the ingredient list.

HOW MUCH DOES MY CHILD NEED?: Fat is essential to support a child's rapid growth since it's a concentrated source of calories. Your baby will nearly triple her birth weight and gain about 10 inches (25 cm) in length by her first birthday, so you'll want to ensure your baby consumes healthy fats at each meal.

All About: Vitamins

WHAT THEY DO: Vitamins perform a wide variety of functions, from forming red blood cells to boosting the immune system to helping release energy from food. They also support the body's metabolic processes. Thirteen vitamins are known to be essential for normal growth, development, and maintenance of our bodies.

TYPES: Vitamins are divided into two categories: fat-soluble and water-soluble.

- The four fat-soluble vitamins are A, D, E, and K. Fat-soluble vitamins are absorbed with the help of fat from foods.
- The water-soluble vitamins are vitamin C and the eight B vitamins: Thiamin (B1), Riboflavin (B2), Niacin (B3), Pantothenic acid (B5), Pyridoxine (B6), Vitamin B12, Biotin (a B vitamin), and Folic acid (a B vitamin).

SOURCES: With the exception of vitamin D, which is produced in the skin when exposed to sunlight, the body cannot manufacture the other 11 vitamins, so you need to get them from the food you eat. All the essential vitamins are found in a wide variety of foods: fruits, berries, vegetables, grains, beans, legumes, dairy, fish and seafood, poultry, and meat.

Most of the B vitamins can be found in whole and fortified grains and cereals, as well as in dairy foods, meat, fish and poultry, some leafy greens, and potatoes.

Vitamin B-12 can be a concern with strict vegetarians who do not eat any foods from animal origin. The only good source is from animals, including meats, poultry, eggs, seafood, and dairy foods.

HOW MUCH DOES MY CHILD NEED?: Only very small amounts of vitamins are needed, but symptoms from vitamin deficiencies may develop if vitamins are lacking in adequate amounts. (See information on individual vitamins in charts on page 193.) On the other hand, when taken in excess, as with supplements, some vitamins may be harmful. According to the American Academy of Pediatrics, healthy children do not need vitamin supplements, provided they have a balanced diet of varied fruits and vegetables, whole-grain complex carbohydrates, fat, and protein.

A GUIDE TO VITAMINS

The following chart provides guidelines for foods that are rich sources of vitamins for infants and toddlers.

VITAMIN	WHAT IT DOES	SOURCES
VITAMIN A	It keeps skin, hair, and nails healthy and helps maintain gums, glands, bones, and teeth. It's necessary for normal vision and bolsters the immune system.	SIX TO ELEVEN MONTHS Carrots and sweet potatoes, butternut squash, red bell peppers, parsley, winter squash, romaine lettuce, broccoli, pumpkin, plantains, butter head lettuce, kale, green bell peppers, green beans, green peas, avocados, okra, rutabagas, and crookneck and acorn squash TWELVE TO TWENTY-FOUR MONTHS Milk and milk products, butter, cheese, eggs, fortified milk, carrots and sweet potatoes, mustard greens, spinach, butternut squash, red bell peppers, parsley, winter squash, beet greens, basil, Romaine lettuce, broccoli, pumpkin, plantains, butter head lettuce, tomatoes, kale, green bell peppers, green beans, green peas, asparagus, avocados, tomatoes, okra, rutabagas, asparagus, Swiss chard, collards, and crookneck and acorn squash **Signs of deficiency:** Night blindness; dry eyes; growth delay in children; dry, rough skin; and low resistance to infection
VITAMIN C (ASCORBIC ACID)	It helps bind cells together, helps heal wounds, and strengthens blood vessel walls.	SIX TO ELEVEN MONTHS Guavas, kiwis, papayas, and cantaloupes; red, orange, yellow, and green bell peppers; parsley; raspberries, honeydew melons, pineapples, blueberries, grapes, and apricots; broccoli, kohlrabi, cauliflower, kale, snow peas, cabbage, and romaine lettuce; plums, cherries, peaches, nectarines, bananas, apples, and pears; and broad beans, rutabagas, butternut squash, potatoes, mixed greens, okra, peas, parsnips, turnips, yams, sweet potatoes and plantains TWELVE TO TWENTY-FOUR MONTHS Guavas, kiwis, papayas, strawberries, oranges, lemons, limes, cantaloupes, grapefruits, and tangerines; red, orange, yellow, and green bell peppers; parsley; mangos, raspberries, honeydew melons, blackberries, star fruit, pineapples, blueberries, grapes, and apricots; broccoli, Brussels sprouts, kohlrabi, cauliflower, kale, snow peas, cabbage, garlic, mustard greens, beet greens, spinach, romaine lettuce, and radishes, watermelon, bananas, cherries, plums, peaches, apples, nectarines, and pears; broad beans, tomatoes, Swiss chard, rutabagas, collard greens, mixed greens (loose leaf lettuce), basil, butternut squash, potatoes, okra, peas, parsnips, turnips, yams, sweet potatoes, plantains, asparagus, and artichokes **Signs of deficiency:** Bleeding gums and loose teeth; bruising; dry, rough skin; slow healing; and appetite loss

VITAMIN	WHAT IT DOES	SOURCES
VITAMIN D	It promotes calcium absorption and builds and maintain bones and teeth.	SIX TO ELEVEN MONTHS Most formulas are fortified with vitamin D. If you are breast-feeding, ask your pediatrician if you need to supplement your baby's diet with vitamin D. TWELVE TO TWENTY-FOUR MONTHS Toddlers who drink vitamin D-fortified whole milk will get an adequate amount of vitamin D. Natural sources include mackerel, salmon, sardines, and egg yolks. Fortified sources include milk and milk products, butter, cheese, and some breakfast cereals. In addition, careful and moderate exposure to sunlight without sun screen is a good source of Vitamin D. **Signs of deficiency:** Thinning and weakening of bones
VITAMIN E	It helps form red blood cells, muscles, and other tissues and prevents cell damage, and preserves fatty acids.	Olive, safflower, soybean, and corn oils; whole grains; leafy vegetables such as Swiss chard, broccoli, spinach, mustard greens, and parsley; avocados; nuts and nut butters; and some seafood **Signs of deficiency:** Blood problems in premature infants; and neurological problems in older children
VITAMIN K	It's needed for normal blood clotting and helps maintain healthy bones.	Green leafy vegetables such as spinach, kale, cabbage, lettuce, broccoli; potatoes; whole grains such as oats, wheat bran; and soy beans **Signs of deficiency:** Excessive bleeding

All About: Minerals

WHAT IT DOES: Although the body needs only small amounts of each mineral, they all play important roles in our bodies. Calcium is the major mineral for our bones and teeth. Iron is vital for our red blood cells and muscles. Other minerals maintain fluid balance, sustain a normal heartbeat, and transmit nerve impulses. Iodine is needed for the thyroid gland. Fluoride is necessary, especially in children, for strong teeth and bones, and it enhances the body's uptake of calcium.

TYPES: Minerals fall into two groups: major and trace minerals.

- The six major minerals are calcium, phosphorus, magnesium, sodium, chloride, and potassium. The last three are known as electrolytes, which are essential for sustaining the body's proper fluid balance.
- The thirteen trace minerals are needed only in small amounts—but they are nutritionally important, especially iron and zinc.

SOURCES: The six major minerals and thirteen trace minerals are found in a wide variety of foods: milk and dairy products, eggs, tofu, seafood, poultry, meat, beans, legumes, nuts and whole grain breads and cereals, and some vegetables.

HOW MUCH DOES MY CHILD NEED?: A varied and balanced diet usually provides adequate amounts of all essential minerals. However, infants and toddlers do have special requirements for iron, zinc, and calcium, which are needed to support the rapid skeletal muscle, bone growth, and expansion of blood volume during the two first years.

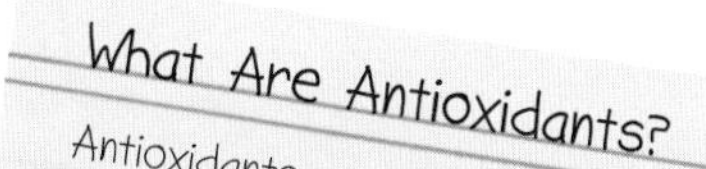

What Are Antioxidants?

Antioxidants are flavor compounds, pigments, or nutrients found in brightly colored foods. The four primary antioxidants are beta-carotene (converted to vitamin A by the body), vitamins C and E, and the mineral selenium. These antioxidants protect our cells from harm caused by free-radicals, or molecules responsible for aging and certain diseases. While free-radicals can damage our cells, antioxidants can help prevent or slow this damage. Antioxidants may also strengthen our immune system and lower the risk of infection.

A GUIDE TO MINERALS

The following charts outline foods that are quality sources of minerals for your infant or toddler. Remember to remove pits and seeds from fruits and vegetables and introduce them appropriately according to your child's age.

MINERAL	WHAT IT DOES	SOURCES
Calcium	It builds bones and teeth and is essential for blood clotting and nerve and muscle function.	SIX TO ELEVEN MONTHS Breast milk, infant formula, and calcium-fortified infant cereal; Cheddar, ricotta, Swiss, mozzarella, and Parmesan cheeses; cottage cheese; yogurt; tofu (processed with calcium sulfate); dried figs; and parsley TWELVE TO TWENTY-FOUR MONTHS Milk, cream, ice cream, yogurt, cheeses, tofu (processed with calcium sulfate), dried figs, halibut, trout, beet greens, collard greens, spinach, basil, and parsley
Iron	It's necessary for the formation of hemoglobin in red blood cells; hemoglobin carries oxygen to every cell in the body.	SIX TO ELEVEN MONTHS Iron-fortified infant formula, iron-fortified infant cereals, egg yolk, lentils and dry beans, soy bean products, dried figs, dates, raisins, prunes, avocados, spinach, parsley, basil, green beans, and green peas TWELVE TO TWENTY-FOUR MONTHS Iron-fortified cereals, beef, pork, lamb, dark meat poultry, lentils, dry beans, soy beans, ground nuts and nut butters, dried figs, dates, raisins, prunes, avocados, Brussels sprouts, green beans, green peas, Swiss chard, beet greens, spinach, parsley, and basil
Zinc	It's essential for normal cell growth, wound healing, and sexual maturation. It is also an essential component in many enzymes.	SIX TO ELEVEN MONTHS Zinc-fortified infant formula, zinc-fortified infant cereals, whole grains (except wheat), rolled oats, Cheddar cheese, ricotta cheese, lentils, split peas, chickpeas, lima beans, green peas, spinach, and parsley TWELVE TO TWENTY-FOUR MONTHS Zinc-fortified cereals, rolled oats, whole grains (except wheat), shellfish, meats and poultry, yogurt, Cheddar cheese, Parmesan cheese, mozzarella cheese, ricotta cheese, lentils, split peas, chickpeas, lima beans, green peas, spinach, parsley, and ground nuts and nut butters

(continued)

MINERAL	WHAT IT DOES	SOURCES
Iodine	It's essential for normal function of the thyroid gland.	Iodized salt, seafood, and seaweed
Fluoride	It strengthens bones and teeth and enhances the body's absorption of calcium.	Fluoridated water and tea
Other Trace Minerals (arsenic, chromium, cobalt, copper, manganese, molybdenum, nickel, selenium, silicon, tin, and vanadium)	They play a role in a variety of metabolic functions.	A balanced diet will provide sufficient amounts of these trace minerals.

Avoiding Iron, Calcium, Zinc, and Iodine Deficiencies

Minerals are critical to sustain an infant's growth. Fortunately, choosing the right foods will ensure your baby gets what he needs.

MINERAL SPOTLIGHT: IRON

Iron plays a major role in a child's development, so it's particularly important that a baby's diet include good sources of the mineral. The natural supply of iron an infant is born with is usually used up by the age of six months. At that time, breast milk and iron-fortified formula are still important sources of iron, but diet becomes a key supplier of this nutrient. Let your pediatrician know you are preparing your own baby food. He may or may not prescribe an iron supplement.

For toddlers over one year old, ¼ to ½ cup (55 to 115 g) iron-fortified cereal a day should provide an adequate amount of iron. Drinking vitamin C–rich juices such as apple or white grape juice or eating vitamin C–rich fruit including peaches, berries, and oranges with iron-fortified baby cereal enhances iron absorption.

After age two, growth rate slows, iron reserves begin to build, and the risk of iron deficiency decreases. Symptoms of iron-deficiency anemia in your baby include fatigue, weakness, and increased susceptibility to infections. If you suspect your child is iron deficient, call your pediatrician.

MINERAL SPOTLIGHT: CALCIUM

Calcium promotes the growth of strong bones and teeth and prevents osteoporosis later in life. Both breast milk and formula provide all of your baby's calcium needs for most of his first year. After that, diet will again play a key role in helping him meet his requirements.

According to the American Academy of Pediatrics, toddlers between the ages of one and three need about 500 milligrams of calcium daily, or the equivalent of two cups of milk or one cup of milk plus one to two ounces of cheese.

Lack of calcium in the diet can cause rickets, a childhood disorder involving softening and weakening of the bones. Always check with a pediatrician if you have any concern about your baby.

MINERAL SPOTLIGHT: ZINC

Zinc is used by the body for growth and development, immune response, neurological function, and reproduction. Healthy, full-term, breastfed babies do not need additional zinc beyond what they get from breast milk, formula, or diet.

Some of the symptoms of mild zinc deficiency in infants and toddlers are diminished appetite, slow growth, increased infections and diarrhea, and a reduced sense of taste and smell. If you are concerned about your baby, check with your pediatrician.

MINERAL SPOTLIGHT: IODINE

At one time in the United States, iodine deficiency disorder (IDD) was a serious problem, jeopardizing children's mental health. Since the introduction of iodized salt, however, it is no longer a concern in this country.

Iodine is also found in seafood and vegetables grown in iodine-rich soil. Breast milk and iodine-fortified infant formulas are the best sources of iodine for infants.

Water For Infant Formula: What's Best?

Pediatricians consider fluoridated tap water safe to use when preparing infant formula since exposure to fluoride during infancy helps prevent tooth decay, but check with your pediatrician for the best recommendation. While all types of infant formulas have low amounts of fluoride, when mixed with tap water, they may contribute fluoride to your baby's diet, increasing his risk for fluorosis, a cosmetic dental issue that leaves faint white marks on both baby teeth and permanent teeth. If you're concerned about fluorosis, you can reduce your baby's exposure to fluoride by alternating tap water with bottled water. Bottled water low in fluoride is labeled "purified," "de-ionized," "de-mineralized," "distilled," or made by reverse osmosis.

All About: Water

WHAT IT DOES: Water is essential to life. It is necessary for digesting food, maintaining proper body temperature, transporting nutrients, eliminating waste products, and lubricating joints.

HOW MUCH DOES MY CHILD NEED?: During an infant's first six months, water isn't necessary, since breast milk or formula provides all the fluid they need. Once your baby starts eating solid food and the requirements for nursing and formula have been met, water can be given from a bottle or cup to quench thirst.

From one year on, your toddler needs 2 cups of milk (16 ounces) a day, after which you can use water if she is still thirsty.

Drink Up! Water That's Safe for Children

Most tap water is safe for both healthy adults and children. The United States has one of the safest water supplies in the world. The Environmental Protection Agency's (EPA's) current drinking water standards are designed to protect children and adults. However, infants' and toddlers' immune systems are not yet fully developed. Consequently, they are more vulnerable to impurities in drinking water. Certain microbes may induce diarrhea and vomiting, which could cause babies to become dehydrated. Young children may also be more susceptible to chemical contaminants (lead, nitrites, nitrates, copper, mercury, barium, cadmium, and pesticides) that affect learning, motor skills, and sex hormones during important stages of growth. Since the water quality varies throughout the country, concerned parents can find out about the safety of their local water by calling the Safe Drinking Water Hotline, 800-426-4791, or the EPA Children's Environmental Health Hotline, 877-590-KIDS.

All About: Sodium

WHAT IT DOES: Sodium, or table salt, maintains fluid balance in the body and helps nerves perform properly.

SOURCES: Salt is found naturally in many foods and water, and processed foods often have salt added as a preservative.

HOW MUCH DOES MY CHILD NEED?: Salt should never be added to the food of babies under twelve months of age. Breast milk and infant formula will provide all the sodium your baby needs. Once a healthy one-year-old starts to eat table food, very small amounts of salt will not be harmful. However, salt is an acquired taste, so use it sparingly. Use spices, herbs, and lemon juice to flavor family recipes if desired, and add just enough salt to bring out the natural flavors without making the food taste salty.

Look for Low-Sodium Foods

Most processed foods have very high levels of sodium, so when feeding your toddler, it's a good idea to check nutrition labels. Look for foods labeled "low sodium" or "reduced sodium." But stay away from "lite" salt; it has been known to cause allergic reactions. In addition, check labels for monosodium glutamate (MSG), a flavor enhancer that can cause allergic reactions and migraines in some people.

All About: Sugar

WHAT IT DOES: Sugar is a source of energy; however, it is devoid of vitamins, minerals, or any other nutrients and is often referred to as providing "empty calories."

TYPES: Sugar, also called sucrose, comes from beets or sugarcane. Molasses is the concentrate that remains after sucrose is extracted from sugarcane. Brown sugar is white sugar crystals that have been coated with molasses. Maple sugar and maple syrup are products of sap from the maple tree, and honey is produced by bees from the nectar of flowers.

SOURCES: Sugars are simple carbohydrates that occur naturally in many foods such as fruit, vegetables, and milk. Refined sugars and other sweeteners are used extensively in processed food. In addition to those used in soft drinks, canned and frozen fruits, breakfast cereals, candy, jams, dairy desserts, fruit drinks, and baked goods, sugar is also found in ketchup, bread, canned vegetables, mustard, salad dressings, and many other unlikely products that we don't think of as being sweet. To make up for the flavor sacrificed by low-fat ingredients, some food manufacturers have increased the sugar content in their products. Consequently, consumption of sugar, honey, and other sweeteners has increased dramatically in the past decade.

HIDDEN SUGARS: Remember that processed foods can contain large amounts of sugar. Be sure to read food labels carefully. The following are different kinds of sugars to watch for in nutrition labels: glucose, dextrose, fructose, sucrose, maltose, lactose, honey, molasses, maple syrup, cane sugar, brown sugar, beet sugar, corn sugar, refined sugar, corn sweetener, corn syrup, high fructose corn syrup, and fruit juice concentrate. A food is high in sugar when one of these sugars appears first or second on the ingredient list.

Honey Warning

The American Academy of Pediatrics recommends that honey not be given to infants younger than twelve months of age. It has been associated with infant botulism, an illness that can be fatal for babies. Honey is often added to bread, jam, crackers, and other baked products, as well as ice cream or yogurt, so read labels carefully.

HOW MUCH DOES MY CHILD NEED?: All sugars, honey, and syrups should be used sparingly. An excess of sugar in a baby's diet can cause diarrhea. Sugar also promotes tooth decay. All sugars are virtually identical nutrition-wise and supply about 4 calories per gram (with the exception of honey, which is higher in calories).

Babies and toddlers naturally love sweets. The challenge for parents is to find the best way to satisfy their child's sweet tooth without jeopardizing oral and general health. Naturally sweet fruits are always the best choice for desserts since they also provide essential vitamins, minerals, and fiber—benefits not provided by most processed cookies, candies, and pastries.

Soft Drinks: Liquid Candy

Carbonated soft drinks have been called liquid candy by many health professionals, and it's easy to see why: A 12-ounce (355 ml) can of soda may contain the equivalent of 10 teaspoons (40 g) of sugar. Not only are carbonated drinks the most common source of empty calories in many children's diets, they also frequently take the place of beneficial beverages in the diet: milk, fruit juices (which should be limited to 4 ounces [120 ml] a day), and water. Plus, chemicals in certain sodas can cause minerals to leach from the bones. In a recent study, findings showed that infants as young as seven months were being given soda on a regular basis, which could explain contributing causes to the current obesity epidemic.

What About Juice?

Juices contain a lot of sugar, so from six months to two years of age, it is preferable to limit the amount of juice a child consumes to four ounces a day. Too much juice can fill small stomachs, leaving insufficient room for a balanced diet. Excessive amounts may cause cramping, diarrhea, and contribute to tooth decay.

However, juice does provide essential vitamins, and it is one of the healthier ways of satisfying your baby's sweet tooth. For six- and seven-month-old babies, juices should be diluted with an equal amount of water. By eight months, your baby may be given full-strength juice, but it's still preferable to dilute it.

When buying juices, look for 100 percent fruit juice—check the label for the words 100 percent pure or 100 percent juice—with no sugar added. This will ensure you are getting only pure fruit juice, not a sweetened juice beverage diluted with water. There are a number of juices fortified with vitamin C made specifically for infants and toddlers. Should you choose to give your child adult juices, be sure they are vitamin C-fortified and that apple juice and cider have been pasteurized to eliminate harmful bacteria.

Steer clear of product names with the words juice cocktail, juice punch, juice drink, juice sparkler, juice blend, or juice beverage since these are terms used for sweetened and diluted juices. And be wary of products labeled "real fruit." They can be misleading, as it means only that the fruit is real, not necessarily that the beverage contains 100 percent fruit juice.

Sweets: Let Them Be the Occasional Treat

We all know that sugar consumption should be limited in both children and adults. But it's important to point out that sweets should not be fanatically denied but rather should be enjoyed occasionally as a treat. In addition, sweets also should not be withheld as a punishment or used as a reward, as that can set up children to become psychologically "addicted" to certain foods, particularly sweets.

All About: Dairy Products and Substitutes

When it comes to dairy products, your options can be overwhelming. But we've simplified everything for you, making the complex simple.

WHOLE COW'S MILK

By the time your baby is one year old, you can start to give him 2 to 3 cups (16 to 24 ounces) of whole milk each day. Whole milk is an important and inexpensive source of the fats, protein, calcium, and vitamins A and D your child needs. All cow's milk given to toddlers and young children should be pasteurized. Instead of giving your toddler a whole cup, which may fill up his little stomach and not leave room for any other food, give him 1⁄4 cup (60 ml) various times throughout the day.

The calcium found in whole cow's milk is most easily absorbed than calcium from other sources. It contains the "good" fats that are important to both infant and toddler development, so it's no surprise pediatricians recommend whole milk for a minimum of the first two to three years of age.

GOAT'S MILK

After twelve months of age, when the digestive system has developed and your baby is eating a healthy diet, goat's milk may be beneficial if cow's milk isn't being well tolerated. Goat's milk contains about 10 grams of fat per 8 ounces (235 ml) compared to 8 to 9 grams in whole cow's milk, and its milk proteins can be easier for a baby to digest. If you choose goat's milk for a one-year-old (or older), be sure it has been pasteurized.

DRIED MILK

There are a number of benefits of dried milk: It is less costly than liquid milk but has the same nutritional value, and it keeps for a long time. However, children up to age two should always drink full-fat milk, and it can be difficult to find dried whole milk; it is usually only available in low-fat and nonfat forms. If you can find dried whole milk (camping outfitters and bakers' suppliers sometimes carry it), by all means, serve it to your child. But you should not offer him dried nonfat or low-fat milk.

MILK SUBSTITUTES

Soy milk (not soy formula) is made from puréed soy beans and water, so it lacks the calcium found in whole cow's milk. Further, soy milk doesn't contain the level of fat, vitamins A and B12, and protein that whole cow's milk does and may even hinder the absorption of calcium due to the phylates it contains, so we don't recommend this option for baby.

Coconut milk is not really milk but the extract pressed from grated coconut. It is very high in calories (552 in 1 cup [235 ml]). It does not have a significant amount of calcium and minimal amounts of iron and vitamin C. Coconut milk has ten times as much saturated fat as whole milk but no cholesterol. Coconut milk should not replace regular milk for toddlers, but its use in Asian recipes, particularly in Thai food, can add variety to the diet.

Rice milk and rice milk products have little nutritional value except for some carbohydrates and a large amount of folate. They are not good substitutes for regular milk, as they lack necessary fat, calcium, protein, vitamin A, and vitamin D. However, it is fine to use rice milk products occasionally as a treat or in smoothies.

OTHER DAIRY PRODUCTS

Whole-milk yogurt, cottage cheese, and ricotta cheese are all high in calcium and can be used liberally in your toddler's diet. Parmesan, mozzarella, and Cheddar cheeses are also excellent sources of calcium and vitamin A. Ice cream, cream, and half-and-half have about the same amount of calcium as milk but almost twice as much fat, cholesterol, and calories as whole milk. They can be used in a toddler's diet, but should be given in moderation. Remember, habits are quickly established but hard to change, so go easy on the high-fat and sweetened dairy products for your child. And keep in mind that once extra calories are not needed, frequent use of cream-based high fat and high cholesterol food should be modified.

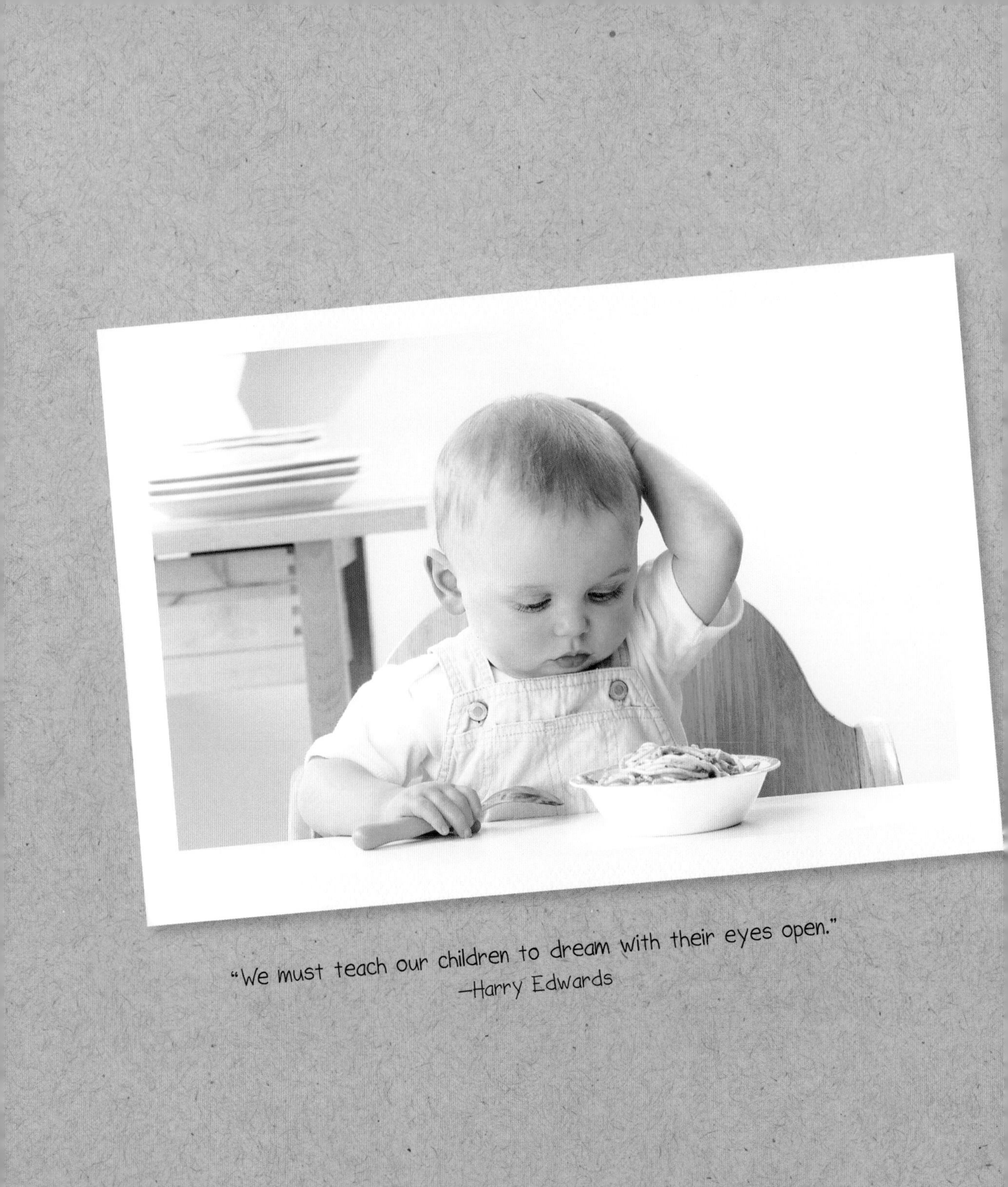

"We must teach our children to dream with their eyes open."
—Harry Edwards

CHAPTER FIVE

Special Considerations

The philosophy of *The Best Homemade Baby Food on the Planet* is built on the premise that the food your child gets accustomed to eating as an infant is the food she'll prefer later in life. While it might seem challenging to keep fast foods, soda, sweets, and other temptations at arms' length, once you establish healthy eating behaviors, your child will prefer natural, fresh meals and snacks as opposed to those with little to no nutritional value.

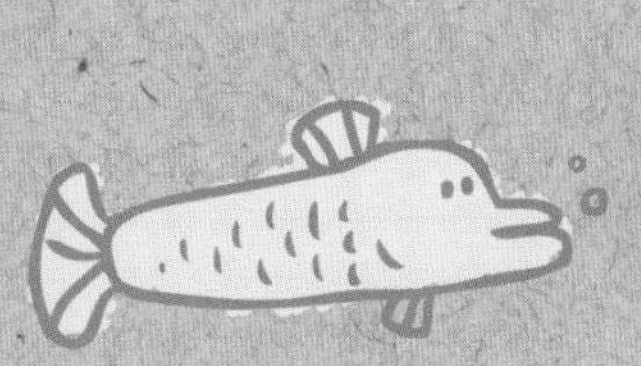

Keeping Weight Problems at Bay

Good nutrition from birth through preschool sets the foundation for healthy habits later in life, but easy access to fast food and junk food can quickly erode these habits. Statistic show that children's eating habits are beginning to mirror those of adult's; almost 25 percent of children ages two to five are overweight or obese in the United States.

During the last decade, there has been much debate and discussion about the dramatic increase in the number of overweight children in the United States. Experts agree that children become overweight for a variety of reasons. The most common reasons are genetic factors, unhealthy food and eating patterns, and lack of physical activity.

While there's not a lot parents can do about the genetic causes of obesity, they can help a child establish healthy exercise and eating habits, and it's precisely these good habits that will offer protection from disease and continue to deliver health benefits for a lifetime.

AVOIDING AND LIMITING FAST FOOD AND JUNK FOOD

If given the choice, children will opt for French fries and ice cream instead of potatoes and yogurt, but this is true only if they have been exposed to these types of meals early and often. So, try to limit trips to the drive-thru, fast food chains, convenience stores, and the snack food aisle in the grocery store. Also limit sugared cereals, pizza, milk shakes, pie, artificially flavored fruit drinks, ice cream, deep-fried chicken, hot dogs, cheeseburgers, soda, and candy.

While cookies or a small piece of cake are just fine for an occasional treat, regular consumption leaves little room for nutrition-dense balanced meals the rest of the day. If you think that your toddler is too heavy, talk to your pediatrician or a registered dietitian who can help you customize a program to meet the special needs of your child.

Nipping Unhealthy Habits in the Bud

The food your child becomes accustomed to eating as a baby is the food she will prefer later in life. Keep in mind, you should not fight, deny, or try to force your child's taste. Her own likes and dislikes will develop naturally from having been given healthy and tasty food at home. Remember, if a child does not acquire a taste for food with little or no nutritional value, she may find it easy to pass them up when she's older.

Understanding Allergies and Food Intolerance: How to Know the Difference

Food intolerance is common among infants and toddlers, but it can be difficult to diagnose. That's why it is important to introduce new foods to your baby one at a time and watch for reactions. If you offer two or more new foods at the same time and there is a reaction, it will be difficult to determine which food caused the problem.

The risk of allergies and food intolerance lessens by the eighth or ninth month and continues to decrease after the first year until the third year, when the risk levels off.

According to the American Academy of Pediatrics, true food allergies, which set the immune system into action, are rare. If you notice a reaction, it is more likely your child is experiencing intolerance to a particular food or ingredient. Keep in mind that allergic reactions don't always happen the first time a food is given, so be aware that your child may develop an allergy to a food he previously tolerated. Consult your pediatrician to correctly identify if a reaction is an intolerance or allergy.

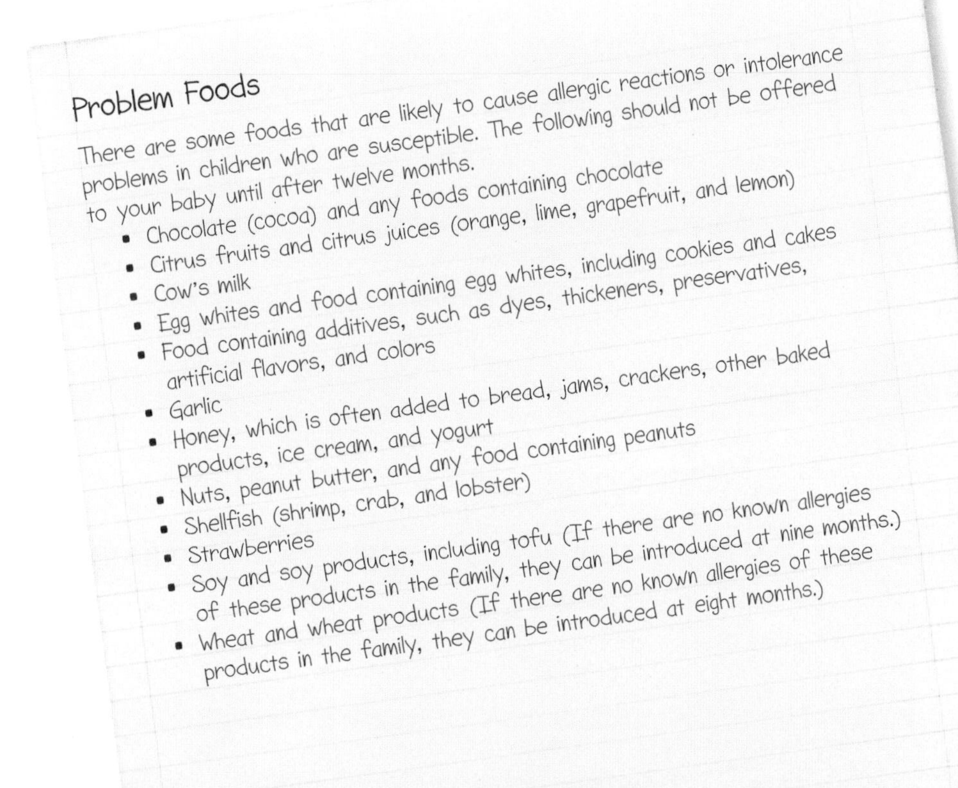

Problem Foods

There are some foods that are likely to cause allergic reactions or intolerance problems in children who are susceptible. The following should not be offered to your baby until after twelve months.

- Chocolate (cocoa) and any foods containing chocolate
- Citrus fruits and citrus juices (orange, lime, grapefruit, and lemon)
- Cow's milk
- Egg whites and food containing egg whites, including cookies and cakes
- Food containing additives, such as dyes, thickeners, preservatives, artificial flavors, and colors
- Garlic
- Honey, which is often added to bread, jams, crackers, other baked products, ice cream, and yogurt
- Nuts, peanut butter, and any food containing peanuts
- Shellfish (shrimp, crab, and lobster)
- Strawberries
- Soy and soy products, including tofu (If there are no known allergies of these products in the family, they can be introduced at nine months.)
- Wheat and wheat products (If there are no known allergies of these products in the family, they can be introduced at eight months.)

If your baby experiences diarrhea, bloating, or gas after eating a new food, immediately stop offering the food. Once you are sure it is intolerance and not an allergy (by checking with your pediatrician), try reintroducing that food a month or two later. If the intolerance recurs, wait until your baby turns one year old before offering that food again.

Diarrhea, skin rashes, hives (itchy welts), wheezing, vomiting, difficult breathing, a runny nose, and tearing eyes are all symptoms of an allergic reaction. If your baby exhibits these symptoms after trying a new food, call your pediatrician immediately. Do not give the food to your baby again until your pediatrician has made a diagnosis.

LACTOSE INTOLERANCE

When the body lacks a needed enzyme (lactase) to digest the natural sugar in milk (lactose), some people may experience lactose intolerance. The most common symptoms are gas, bloating, and diarrhea. Infants are born with high levels of lactase, but by age three or four, it has decreased, especially in people of Asian, African, southern European, and Native American ancestry. However, not all lactase-deficient people are lactose intolerant.

By age three or four, many children with lactose intolerance are also intolerant of soy products. Some, however, have only a partial intolerance and can handle milk and dairy products so long as only small amounts are served with food. Aged cheeses and yogurts are usually acceptable because the lactose is broken down during the aging process.

Reduced-lactose and lactose-free milk is now readily available, as are lactase enzyme products that can be added to milk and dairy foods to make lactose digestible. Check with your pediatrician before giving this milk to your child.

HIGH-RISK CHILDREN

The American Academy of Pediatrics recommends the following to prevent or delay food allergies in infants at high risk, such as those with a family history food of allergies.

- Breast-feed exclusively for the first six months or use a low-allergenic formula (no cow's milk or soy protein) as recommended by your pediatrician.
- While nursing, eliminate nuts, peanuts, eggs, and milk from your diet.
- Delay the introduction of solid foods until after six months of age.
- Delay the introduction of cow's milk until age one, eggs until age two, and peanuts, nuts, and fish until age three.

Oral Health: Building Good Habits for Healthy Teeth

Care and cleaning of your child's teeth is a collaboration between you and your pediatric dentist, but there really is a lot you can do on your own to prevent potential oral health problems before they occur.

TEETHING

There is a wide variation in the age that babies cut their first teeth, but the first teeth usually appear between five and seven months. Teething often causes problems like sore and painful gums, which may make babies cranky and irritable, reduce their appetite, or even cause diaper rash. Since so many teeth are cut during the first two years, there may be many trying times.

A baby often has an elevated temperature during teething. A fever of 100°F (38°C) or higher, however, requires a call to the pediatrician. If feverish, give your baby plenty of liquids. It is important to get the fever down as quickly as possible, but do not give him any medicine without your pediatrician's advice. If your baby has diarrhea, cut out fruits and fruit juice until symptoms have disappeared, but do not eliminate or decrease breast milk or formula. Plain, puréed boiled rice can also be helpful.

For babies, rubbing the gums with a clean finger may ease some of the discomfort, and clean and frozen washcloths or terrycloth may be nice for them to chew on. Your baby may try to put hard objects in her mouth, so be careful that the object is not something she might choke on. Extra love, patience, and cuddling will be needed at this time.

For toddlers, frozen berries, fruits, and some vegetables (cut into small pieces to prevent choking) and other cooked and frozen foods like mini waffles are popular during periods of teething, as they soothe swollen gums. If you feel your child might need medication for relief, ask your pediatrician.

CAVITY PREVENTION

A balanced diet is not only important to infants' and toddlers' general health, but also for their dental health. Baby and toddler tooth decay had until recently been blamed primarily on baby bottle tooth decay syndrome, cavities developed from allowing a child to drink from bottles of juice or milk while falling asleep, which can cause the liquid to pool in the mouth. A broader viewpoint now includes the following other causes of tooth decay and methods of prevention:

- Start early with good nutrition, eating habits, and oral hygiene.
- Don't dip pacifiers in sugar, honey, or juice. (Never give honey to a baby less than a year old under any circumstances.)
- Limit fruit juices to ½ cup (120 ml) daily.
- Do not offer juice or other sweet liquids in a bottle—only in a cup. If you must give your baby something to suck on at bedtime for comfort, use only water or a pacifier.
- Wipe your baby's gums with a soft, wet washcloth to remove harmful bacteria.
- When your baby has a few teeth, either brush them with a soft-bristle brush or wipe them off after meals with a wet piece of gauze.
- Pay an early visit to a pediatric dentist.

Between six and twelve months of age, your baby will generally cut about eight teeth. These primary teeth are important for chewing food, speech, and good appearance. Baby teeth also help reserve space in the jaws for permanent teeth—all significant reasons for keeping them healthy. As soon as the teeth break through, clean them daily with a damp cloth, gauze pad, or soft baby brush. Use only fresh water, no toothpaste. Daily cleaning is essential, as this is the time when solids and juices are added to the diet.

Oral bacteria feed on sugar and starches that are left on the teeth for more than 20 minutes, producing acids that destroy tooth enamel and cause cavities. Foods that tend to cling to baby teeth include sugary foods and high-starch snacks, such as dried fruit, crackers, breadsticks, and teething biscuits. Eating Cheddar, Monterey Jack, or Swiss cheese immediately after sugary and high-starch foods may counteract some of the negative effects but not as thoroughly as cleaning the teeth.

If your water supply is not fluoridated and the natural fluoride content of your water is low, your pediatrician may prescribe a fluoride supplement around six months. By your baby's first birthday, visit a pediatric dentist and ask for a demonstration and information on proper brushing techniques.

Toddlers are not developmentally ready to brush their teeth by themselves yet, but between eighteen months and two years, start teaching your toddler to spit out toothpaste. So long as it is not swallowed, use a pea-sized amount of fluoride toothpaste on the toothbrush and guiding her hand, help her brush her teeth. Training toothpaste without fluoride, which is safe to swallow, is also available for toddlers.

Fluoride, a trace mineral present in varying concentrations in soil and water, plays an important role in the maintenance of healthy teeth and bones. It contributes to the growth of new enamel and also strengthens it, making the teeth more resistant to decay.

According to the American Dental Association, research shows that fluoride reduces children's cavities by up to 50 percent. As a direct result of water fluoridation and over-the-counter fluoride products, half of all children entering first grade today have never had a single cavity, compared with 36 percent in 1980 and 28 percent in the early 1970s. Note that research in areas where the drinking water is naturally rich in fluoride has confirmed the safety of fluoride in the water supply. Virtually all major health organizations endorse and support the use of fluoride as an important tool in promoting dental health.

Last, try not to give your child sugar-rich foods that stick to the teeth, such as mints, lollipops, or hard candy. Avoid soft, sticky sweets such as toffee, fruit leather, and dried fruits (unless soaked and cooked). Instead of sweet snacks, offer cheese, raw vegetables, plain yogurt, or fresh fruit. Variety, moderation, and attention to healthful between-meal snacks will benefit oral and general health.

Diaper Rash and Teething?

Diaper rash, which can be linked to teething, can be kept to a minimum by changing your baby as soon as he becomes wet or soiled. A diaper rash ointment makes a soothing skin barrier. Fresh air and a little sunshine also promote healing.

Fish and Shellfish

Many parents and caregivers are confused about the risks and benefits of feeding seafood to infants, but a January 2009 report from the Food and Drug Administration set the record straight: Fish and shellfish are valuable parts of a healthy diet. They provide high-quality protein and are the most important sources of omega-3 fatty acids, which are essential for normal brain development and heart health. Fish has even acquired the nickname "brain food" for its beneficial effects on cognition and memory. Recent research has also shown that omega-3 fatty acids enhance visual acuity and cognitive and motor skills in children and may even reduce pre-term labor and post-partum depression.

While experts recommend that you introduce fish after your child's first birthday, advice about seafood consumption varies from country to country. If you lived in Asia, for example, or a Scandinavian country where fish is a diet staple, your baby would probably be eating fish before eating meat or chicken. However, in the United States, it's customary to introduce fin fish like tuna and salmon and shellfish including shrimp and crab after a baby has accepted both puréed fruits, vegetables, strained meats, and poultry.

While ocean fish do contain trace amounts of mercury, The U.S. National Oceanic & Atmospheric Administration (USOAA) reports that the mercury issue has been overstated and confusion about mercury and fish has done a great public disservice; no single person in the United States has ever experienced mercury poisoning from normal fish consumption because the FDA's guidelines regarding fish consumption and mercury are the most stringent in the world. Health experts would agree that the real problem is that children don't eat enough seafood.

So, what seafood should you choose? The Institute of Medicine (IOM) has some very simple advice for pregnant and nursing moms as well as young children up to age 12. Enjoy two to three servings (about 12 ounces [340 g]) of a variety of seafood every week, of which up to six ounces can be albacore tuna. (Tuna mercury levels can be different based on the type of tuna and where it was caught. Choose Chunk Light more often than Albacore.) And avoid shark, swordfish, king mackerel, and tilefish since these are known to have the most mercury.

"Fishing" for Great Menu Ideas?

Looking for seafood suggestions for tonight's dinner? Below is a comprehensive shopping list to get you started.

LOWEST MERCURY FISH

- Anchovies
- Butterfish
- Calamari (squid)
- Catfish
- Caviar (farmed)
- Clams
- Crab (king)
- Crawfish/crayfish
- Flounder
- Haddock
- Hake
- Herring
- Lobster (spiny/rock)
- Oysters
- Perch (ocean)
- Pollock
- Salmon
- Sardines
- Scallops
- Shad
- Shrimp
- Sole
- Sturgeon (farmed)
- Tilapia
- Trout (freshwater)
- Whitefish

LOW MERCURY FISH

- Carp
- Cod
- Crab (blue)
- Crab (dungeness)
- Crab (snow)
- Herring
- Mahi Mahi
- Monkfish
- Perch (freshwater)
- Skate
- Snapper
- Tuna (canned, chunk light)
- Tuna (fresh Pacific albacore)

Chart obtained from the Natural Resource Defense Council (NRDC); data obtained by the FDA and the EPA.

Choking

Choking is a very real hazard to children under the age of three. Children should be constantly supervised while they are eating. In addition, don't let your toddler eat while running or playing and teach him to finish each mouthful before speaking. And it is not a good idea to allow your toddler to eat in the car; if he should choke, you may not be able to safely stop the car to help him.

Be careful with firm or slippery foods like hot dogs, hard candy, peanuts, cherries, cherry tomatoes, and grapes; they may be swallowed before they are fully chewed, get lodged in the throat, and cause choking. This can also happen with small, dry, or hard foods that are difficult to chew, like popcorn, potato and corn chips, nuts, seeds, small pieces of raw carrot, or large wads of melted cheese. Some common sticky or tough foods like peanut butter, tough meat, and uncooked raisins or other dried fruit can also easily lodge in the throat and block the airway.

CHOKING PREVENTION

Follow these guidelines when feeding your child to minimize the risk of choking:

- Cook food until it is soft enough to easily pierce with a fork.
- Cut food into small pieces or thin slices small enough for easy chewing.
- Cut round foods, such as hot dogs or cooked carrots, into short strips rather than round pieces.
- Cut grapes in half and remove seeds, if any.
- Cut cherries in half and remove pits.
- Cut cherry tomatoes in quarters.
- Grind or mash and moisten food for young babies.
- Remove all bones.

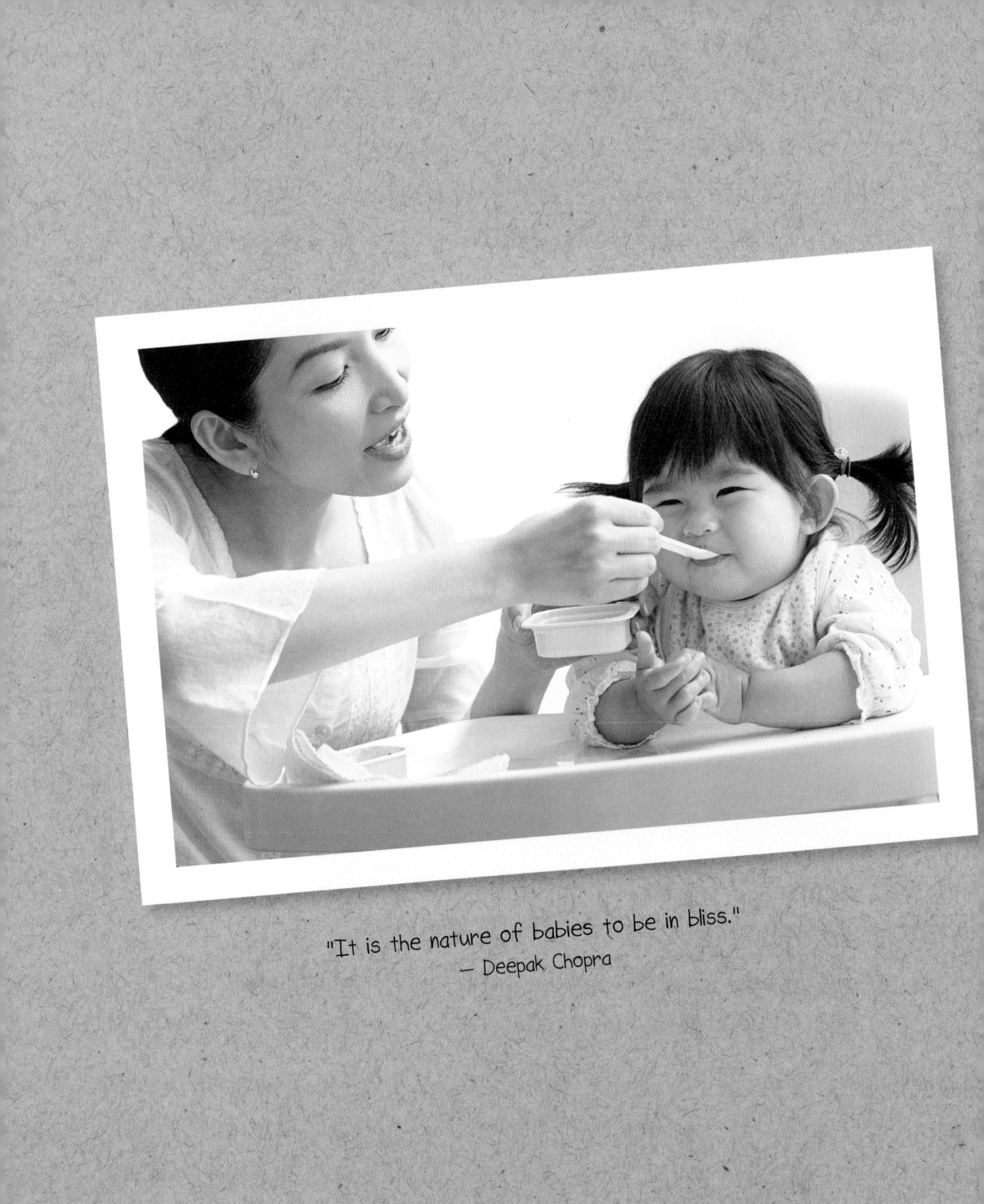

"It is the nature of babies to be in bliss."
— Deepak Chopra

CHAPTER SIX

Resources and References

KITCHEN EQUIVALENT CHART

This handy chart will help you in the kitchen, especially when preparing small amounts of food for baby.

A PINCH	= 1/8 teaspoon or less		
A DASH	= a few drops		
1 TABLESPOON	= 3 teaspoons	= 1/2 ounce	
2 TABLESPOONS	= 1/8 cup	= 1 ounce	
4 TABLESPOONS	= 1/4 cup	= 2 ounces	
5 TABLESPOONS + 1 TEASPOON	= 1/3 cup		
8 TABLESPOONS	= 4 ounces	= 1/2 cup	= 1/4 pound
16 TABLESPOONS	= 8 ounces	= 1 cup	= 1/2 pint
2 CUPS = 16 OUNCES	= 1 pint		
4 CUPS = 2 PINTS	= 1 quart		
16 CUPS = 4 QUARTS	= 1 gallon		

Sources

Aiyer HS, Vadhanam MV, Stoyanova R, Caprio GD, Clapper ML, Gupta RC. Dietary berries and ellagic acid prevent oxidative DNA damage and modulate expression of DNA repair genes. *International Journal of Molecular Sciences*. 2008; 9:327-341.

Agostoni, Carlo, Enrica Riva, Marcello Giovannini. Dietary "Fiber in Weaning Foods of Young Children." *Pediatrics*. November 1995; 96:1002-1005.

American Academy of Pediatrics. "Calcium Requirements of Infants, Children, and Adolescents." *Pediatrics*. November 1999; 104 (no 5): 1152-1157.

American Dietetic Association. "Eat Right Nutrition Tips." Available at: www.eatright.org/Public/content.aspx?id=206. Accessed May 25, 2010.

American Dietetic Association. Position of the American Dietetic Association: Dietary guidance for healthy children 2 to 11 years. *J Am Diet Assoc*. January 1999; 99 (no 1): 1046-1047.

American Dietetic Association. "Promoting and Supporting Breastfeeding." *J Am Diet Assoc*. 2009;109:1926-1942.

American Dietetic Association. "Individual, Family, School, and Community-based Intervention Programs for Pediatric Overweight." *J Am Diet Assoc*. 2006; 106: 925-945.

American Dietetic Association. "Vegetarian Diets." *J Am Diet Assoc*. 2009; 109: 1266-1282.

American Heart Association. "Dietary Recommendations for Healthy Children." Available at: www.americanheart.org/presenter.jhtml?identifier=4575. Accessed May 25, 2010.

American Heart Association. "Fat." Available at: www.americanheart.org/presenter.jhtml?identifier=4582. Accessed May 25, 2010.

American Heart Association. "Nutrition and Children." *Circulation*. 1997; 95 (no 9): 2332-2333.

Birch, Leann L., Jennifer O. Fisher. "Development of Eating Behaviors Among Children and Adolescents." *Pediatrics*. March 1998; 101 (no 3): 539-549.

Cox, Dana R., MS, RD; Jean D. Skinner, PhD, RD; Betty Ruth Carruth, PhD, RD. A food Variety Index for Toddlers (VIT): development and application. *J Am Diet Assoc*. December 1997;97 (no 12): 1382-1386.

Dennison, B.A. Fruit juice consumption by infants and children: a review. *Journal of the American College of Nutrition*. October 1996; 15 (issue 5): 4S-11S.

Environmental Protection Agency. "Children and Drinking Water Standards." Available at: www.epa.gov/safewater/kids/kidshealth/booklet_text.html. Accessed May 25, 2010.

Fisher, Edward A., MD, PhD, MPH; Linda Van Horn, PhD, RD; Henry C McGill, MD. "Nutrition and Children: A Statement for Healthcare Professionals from the Nutrition Committee, American Heart Association." *Circulation*. 1997; 95: 2332-2333.

Fitzsimons, Dina, Johanna Dwyer, Carole Palmer, Linda Boyd. Nutrition and oral health guidelines for pregnant women, infants, and children. *J Am Diet Assoc*. February 1998; 98 (no 2): 182-189.

Forgac, Marilyn T., MS, RD. Timely Statement of the American Dietetic Association: Dietary guidance for healthy children. *ADA Reports*. March 1995; 95 (no 3): 370.

Infants' food allergies rarer than parents believe. *J Allergy Clin Immunol*. May 2006. Available at www.medicineonline.com/news/12/4778/Infants-food-allergies-rarer-than-parents-believe.html. Accessed May 25, 2010.

Isolauri E, Arvola T, Sütas Y, Salminen S. Probiotics in the management of atopic eczema. *Clin Exp Allergy*. 2000; 30: 1605-1610.

Jacobson, Michael F., PhD. "Liquid Candy: How Soft Drinks are Harming Americans' Health." Center for Science in the Public Interest. Available at: www.cspinet.org/sodapop/liquid_candy.htm. Accessed May 25, 2010.

McBride, Judy. "What Americans Eat—For Better, For Worse." *Food & Nutrition Research Briefs*. April 1995. Available at: www.ars.usda.gov/is/np/fnrb/fnrb495.htm#eat. Accessed May 25, 2010.

Mennella, J.A., G.K. Beachamp. Early flavor experiences: research update. *Nutritional Revue*. July 1998; 56 (no 7): 205-211.

Murphy, Anne S., PhD, RD; June P. Youatt, PhD; Sharon L. Hoerr, PhD, RD; Carol A. Sawyer, PhD, RD; Sandra L Andrews PhD, RD. Kindergarten students' food preferences are not consistent with their knowledge of the Dietary Guidelines. *J Am Diet Assoc*. February 1995; 95 (no 2): 219-223.

National Institutes of Health. "Helping Your Overweight Child." *NIH Publication*. January 1997; (no 97): 4096. Available at: http://win.niddk.nih.gov/publications/over_child.htm. Accessed May 25, 2010.

National Institutes of Health. "Statistics Related to Overweight and Obesity." *NIH Publication*. July 1996; (no 96): 4158. Available at: http://win.niddk.nih.gov/statistics/index.htm. Accessed May 25, 2010.

Nicklas, Theresa A. Dietary Trends Among Children. Based on Dietary studies of children: The Bogalusa Heart Study experience. *J Am Diet Assoc*. February 1995 ; 95 (no 2).

Nicklas, Theresa A., PhD; Rosanne P. Farris, MS; Leann Myers, MS; Gerald S. Berenson, MD. Dietary fiber intake of children and young adults: The Bogalusa Heart Study. *J Am Diet Assoc.* February 1995; 95 (no 2).

NIHCM Foundation. "Obesity in Young Children: Impact and Intervention." *NIHCM Obesity Brief.* August 2004. Available at: www.nihcm.org/~nihcmor/pdf/OYCbrief.pdf. Accessed May 25, 2010.

Picciano, Mary Frances, Lois D. McBean, Virginia A. Stallings. How to grow a healthy child: a conference report. *Nutrition Today.* January 1999; 34: 6.

Ross, Emma. Study: "Soft Drinks Lead to Obesity." Associated Press. February 15, 2001.

Saldanha, Leila G., PhD, RD. "Fiber in the Diet of US Children: Results of National Surveys." *Pediatrics.* November 1995; 96.

Saltos, Etta, PhD., Shanthy Bowman, PhD. Dietary Guidance on Sodium: Should we take it with a grain of salt? *Nutrition Insights.* USDA Center of Nutrition Policy and Promotion. May 1997. Available at: www.cnpp.usda.gov/Publications/NutritionInsights/insight3.pdf. Accessed May 25, 2010.

Sicherer SH, Sampson HA. Food allergy. *J Allergy Clin Immunol.* 2006; 117 (2 Suppl Mini-Primer): S470-S475.

Skinner, Jean D., PhD, RD; Betty Ruth Carruth, PhD, RD; Kelly S. Houck, MS; Frances Coletta, PhD, RD; Richard Cotter, PhD; Dana Ott, PhD; and Max McLeod, MS. Longitudinal study of nutrient and food intakes of infants aged 2 to 24 months. *J Am Diet Assoc.* May 1997; 97 (no 5).

Smith, M.M., and F. Lifshitz. Excess fruit juice consumption as a contributing factor in nonorganic failure to thrive. *Pediatrics.* March 1994; 93 (no 3): 438–43.

Stallone, Daryth D., Ph.D., M.P.H., and Michael F. Jacobson, Ph.D. Cheating Babies: "Nutritional Quality and Cost of Commercial Baby Food." *CSPI Reports.* Available at: www.cspinet.org/reports/cheat1.html. Accessed May 25, 2010.

Stedronsky, Frances M., MBA, MA. Child Nutrition and Health Campaign: A member update. *J Am Diet Assoc.* June 1998; 98 (no 7).

Stehlin, Dori. "Feeding Baby Nature and Nurture." *FDA Consumer.* U.S. Food and Drug Administration, September 1990, updated March 1991.

Tsuda, T., Regulation of adipocyte function by anthocyanins; possibility of preventing the metabolic syndrome. *J Agric Food Chem.* 2008; 56 (3): 642-6.

U.S. Department of Agriculture. "Dietary Guidelines for Americans." Available at www.mypyramid.gov/guidelines/index.html. Accessed May 25, 2010.

U.S. Department of Agriculture. "Focus on Ground Beef." October 2009. Available at: www.fsis.usda.gov/Fact_Sheets/ground_beef_and_food_safety/index.asp. Accessed May 25, 2010.

U.S. Department of Agriculture. "Focus on Chicken." April 2006. Available at: www.fsis.usda.gov/Fact_Sheets/Chicken_Food_Safety_Focus/index.asp. Accessed May 25, 2010.

U.S. Department of Agriculture, "What and Where our Children Eat"—1994 Nationwide Survey Results. news release. April 18, 1996. Available at: www.usda.gov/news/releases/1996/04/0197. Accessed May 25, 2010.

U.S. Department of Agriculture, Agricultural Research Service. "Making Calcium More Available." *Food & Nutrition Research Briefs,* January 2002. Available at: www.ars.usda.gov/is/np/fnrb/fnrb102.htm. Accessed May 25, 2010.

U.S. Department of Agriculture, Center for Nutrition Policy and Promotion. Is fruit juice consumption dangerous for children? *Nutrition Insights.* March 1997. Available at: www.cnpp.usda.gov/Publications/NutritionInsights/Insight1.pdf. Accessed May 25, 2010.

U.S. Food and Drug Administration. "Water: New Trends, New Rules." *FDA Consumer.* June 1991.

U.S. Food and Drug Administration. "What You Need to Know About Mercury and Shellfish." March 2004. Available at: www.fda.gov/Food/FoodSafety/Product-SpecificInformation/Seafood/FoodbornePathogensContaminants/Methylmercury/ucm115662.htm. Accessed May 25, 2010.

Whitlock E, Williams RG, Smith P, Shipman S. Screening and interventions for childhood overweight: A summary of evidence for the U.S. Preventive Services Task Force. *Pediatrics.* 2005; 116: 125-144.

Wang SY, Lin HS. Antioxidant activity in fruits and leaves of blackberry, raspberry, and strawberry varies with cultivar and developmental stage. *J Agric Food Chem.* 2000; 48: 140-6.

ACKNOWLEDGMENTS

No writer works alone, so I'd like to thank those whose experience, support, and knowledge helped make this book a reality.

I'd like to thank my agent and long-time friend, Linda Konner, for believing in me and my ability to write this book. I'd also like to thank Karin Knight, who was the best co-author I could have ever hoped for.

I owe a debt of gratitude to my talented editor, Amanda Waddell, for her intelligent editing, for helping me bring my vision of the book to life, and for providing me with an education in publishing along the way. Thanks also to Shannon K. LeMay-Finn, for keeping track of the mind-boggling details during the editing process, and a note of thanks to all my friends for their encouragement and moral support when I could not face another day and yet another purée.

I am beyond grateful to Erin Lane at Beaba for her enthusiastic support of the book when it was just a concept and for providing us with such beautiful products for our photo shoot.

My most generous thanks to Richard for his patience and cheerleading, which made long, long nights (holidays and weekends) at my computer a bit less painful. And last but not least, I offer my deepest, heart-felt gratitude to my mother and father, for each one has given me a particular gift by their example.

—Tina Ruggiero

ABOUT THE AUTHORS

Karin Knight, R.N., is co-author of the best-selling book *The Baby Cookbook* and *1-2-3 Cook for Me*. Before turning cooking into an occupation, she spent twenty-five years working as a registered nurse. She currently resides in Montana with her husband.

Tina Ruggiero, M.S., R.D., L.D., is a sought-after nutritionist, spokesperson, and author. Fondly called the "Gourmet Nutritionist," Tina is heard on TV and radio, and her writing has appeared in magazines such as *Family, Men's Health*, and *First for Women*. Tina is president and founder of her own nutrition consulting firm where she helps both corporations and consumers. She is also a nutrition correspondent for NBC's syndicated television show Daytime where she is seen regularly by millions of viewers around the nation. Her blog, www.voiceofreason.net, is often cited in magazines, newspapers, and on the Internet for its reliable, accurate, and inspiring content.

"Look at What We've Made!": Feedback Chart

Use this section as a guide to track all the delicious meals you've created to nourish and delight your baby. Years from now, it will be a joy to review these pages and remind your not-so-little one that, once upon time, *Puréed Carrots with Pretty Pears* really was her favorite meal!

RECIPE	DATE MADE	BABY STAR RATING (FILL IN THE STARS!)	NOTES (e.g., Any recipe adjustments or variations made?, Was this served on its own or with other items?, Recipe good for batch and freeze?)	MAKE AGAIN?
SIX MONTHS				
Mighty Mouthful Rice Cereal (Page 28)		☆☆☆☆☆		○ Yes ○ No
Baby's First Oatmeal (Page 28)		☆☆☆☆☆		○ Yes ○ No
Perfect Apple Pureé (Page 29)		☆☆☆☆☆		○ Yes ○ No
Sweet Pear Purée (Page 29)		☆☆☆☆☆		○ Yes ○ No
Ready, Set, Go Avocado Purée (Page 30)		☆☆☆☆☆		○ Yes ○ No
Best Banana Sauté (Page 30)		☆☆☆☆☆		○ Yes ○ No
Double Whammy Banan-y (Page 32)		☆☆☆☆☆		○ Yes ○ No
Perfectly Paired Fruit and Grain Oatmeal (Page 32)		☆☆☆☆☆		○ Yes ○ No
Kiss the Cook Pear-Potato Purée (Page 33)		☆☆☆☆☆		○ Yes ○ No
Potassium-Powered Potato-Banana Purée (Page 33)		☆☆☆☆☆		○ Yes ○ No
Baby's Favorite Barley Cereal (Page 34)		☆☆☆☆☆		○ Yes ○ No
Oh So Sweet Potato Purée (Page 34)		☆☆☆☆☆		○ Yes ○ No
Apple-a-Day Oatmeal (Page 36)		☆☆☆☆☆		○ Yes ○ No
Yummy Apple-Pear Purée (Page 36)		☆☆☆☆☆		○ Yes ○ No
More Green Peas Purée, Please! (Page 39)		☆☆☆☆☆		○ Yes ○ No

RECIPE	DATE MADE	BABY STAR RATING (FILL IN THE STARS!)	NOTES	MAKE AGAIN?
SEVEN MONTHS				
Zoom Zoom Zucchini (Page 43)		☆☆☆☆☆		○ Yes ○ No
Sunrise Squash Purée (Page 43)		☆☆☆☆☆		○ Yes ○ No
Creamy Butternut Squash Purée (Page 44)		☆☆☆☆☆		○ Yes ○ No
A Is for Acorn Squash Purée (Page 44)		☆☆☆☆☆		○ Yes ○ No
Wee-licious Potato (Page 46)		☆☆☆☆☆		○ Yes ○ No
Bun-in-the-Oven Baked Potato (Page 46)		☆☆☆☆☆		○ Yes ○ No
No-Cook Prune Purée (Page 47)		☆☆☆☆☆		○ Yes ○ No
Power-Packed Prunes (Page 47)		☆☆☆☆☆		○ Yes ○ No
Super P! No-Cook Purée (Page 48)		☆☆☆☆☆		○ Yes ○ No
Fuzzy Peach Purée (Page 48)		☆☆☆☆☆		○ Yes ○ No
Plum Good Purée (Page 49)		☆☆☆☆☆		○ Yes ○ No
Peachy Plum (Page 49)		☆☆☆☆☆		○ Yes ○ No
Fuss-Free Pumpkin and Banana Purée (Page 50)		☆☆☆☆☆		○ Yes ○ No
Peach and Banana Whip (Page 50)		☆☆☆☆☆		○ Yes ○ No
Prune-Apple-Banana Smoothie (Page 52)		☆☆☆☆☆		○ Yes ○ No
Peachy-Keen Banana Purée (Page 52)		☆☆☆☆☆		○ Yes ○ No
A to B Apple-Butternut Squash Purée (Page 53)		☆☆☆☆☆		○ Yes ○ No
Green Pea and Potato Garden Purée (Page 53)		☆☆☆☆☆		○ Yes ○ No

RECIPE	DATE MADE	BABY STAR RATING (FILL IN THE STARS!)	NOTES	MAKE AGAIN?
EIGHT MONTHS				
Naturally Sweet Apricot Purée (Page 56)		☆☆☆☆☆		○ Yes ○ No
Four-Fruit Compote (Page 56)		☆☆☆☆☆		○ Yes ○ No
Bright Eyes Mashed Carrots (Page 58)		☆☆☆☆☆		○ Yes ○ No
Puréed Carrots with Pretty Pears (Page 58)		☆☆☆☆☆		○ Yes ○ No
Any Way You Please Potato and Peas (Page 59)		☆☆☆☆☆		○ Yes ○ No
Orange You Cute Carrots and Sweet Potato (Page 59)		☆☆☆☆☆		○ Yes ○ No
My First Cheese, Please! (Page 60)		☆☆☆☆☆		○ Yes ○ No
Better-for-Baby Sweet Potato "Fries" (Page 60)		☆☆☆☆☆		○ Yes ○ No
Buttered with Love Green Beans (Page 62)		☆☆☆☆☆		○ Yes ○ No
Mighty Tasty Blueberry and Pear Mash (Page 62)		☆☆☆☆☆		○ Yes ○ No
Basmati Baby Rice (Page 63)		☆☆☆☆☆		○ Yes ○ No
Comfy and Cozy Rice and Apricot Pudding (Page 63)		☆☆☆☆☆		○ Yes ○ No
Positively Perfect Pumpkin and Pears (Page 64)		☆☆☆☆☆		○ Yes ○ No
Color Me Orange Carrot-Potato Purée (Page 64)		☆☆☆☆☆		○ Yes ○ No
Creamy Cottage Cheese and Carrot Purée (Page 66)		☆☆☆☆☆		○ Yes ○ No
Bananas in the Snow (Page 67)		☆☆☆☆☆		○ Yes ○ No
Blueberry and Banana Breakfast (Page 67)		☆☆☆☆☆		○ Yes ○ No
Summertime Watermelon Mash (Page 68)		☆☆☆☆☆		○ Yes ○ No

RECIPE	DATE MADE	BABY STAR RATING (FILL IN THE STARS!)	NOTES	MAKE AGAIN?
That's Beta-Carotene on My Bib! Carrots with Apricots (Page 68)		☆☆☆☆☆		○ Yes ○ No
Blueberry Cottage Cheese with Ease (Page 70)		☆☆☆☆☆		○ Yes ○ No
A-OK Puréed Carrots with Apple (Page 70)		☆☆☆☆☆		○ Yes ○ No
NINE MONTHS				
Happy Potato with Hard-Cooked Egg Yolk (Page 73)		☆☆☆☆☆		○ Yes ○ No
Good Golly Green Beans with Carrot and Apple (Page 73)		☆☆☆☆☆		○ Yes ○ No
Baby's Favorite Puréed Papaya (Page 74)		☆☆☆☆☆		○ Yes ○ No
Easy-Peasy Prune and Papaya Purée (Page 74)		☆☆☆☆☆		○ Yes ○ No
Creamy Broccoli for Baby (Page 75)		☆☆☆☆☆		○ Yes ○ No
Incredible Cauliflower Purée (Page 75)		☆☆☆☆☆		○ Yes ○ No
Little Bunny's Favorite Cauliflower and Carrot (Page 76)		☆☆☆☆☆		○ Yes ○ No
Sweet Omelet Surprise (Page 76)		☆☆☆☆☆		○ Yes ○ No
Egg-cellent Fried Rice (Page 77)		☆☆☆☆☆		○ Yes ○ No
Yummy in My Tummy Banana-Yogurt Puddin' (Page 77)		☆☆☆☆☆		○ Yes ○ No
Triple-Tasty Avocado, Cantaloupe, and Yogurt (Page 78)		☆☆☆☆☆		○ Yes ○ No
Avocado and Peach Mash with Papaya Nectar (Page 78)		☆☆☆☆☆		○ Yes ○ No
Yummy Yummy Carrot-Papaya Yogurt (Page 79)		☆☆☆☆☆		○ Yes ○ No
Lucky Peas, Lucky Me! (Page 79)		☆☆☆☆☆		○ Yes ○ No

RECIPE	DATE MADE	BABY STAR RATING (FILL IN THE STARS!)	NOTES	MAKE AGAIN?
Baby's First Chicken with Corn and Potatoes (Page 80)		☆☆☆☆☆		○ Yes ○ No
Lovely Little Pasta Soup (Page 80)		☆☆☆☆☆		○ Yes ○ No
Chicken with Sweet Potatoes (Page 82)		☆☆☆☆☆		○ Yes ○ No
Highchair Haute Chicken with Peaches (Page 83)		☆☆☆☆☆		○ Yes ○ No
Dreamy Creamy Spinach (Page 83)		☆☆☆☆☆		○ Yes ○ No
Broccoli Au Gratin (Page 84)		☆☆☆☆☆		○ Yes ○ No
Chicken in the Grass (Page 84)		☆☆☆☆☆		○ Yes ○ No
Sweet Potato and Cauliflower Purée (Page 85)		☆☆☆☆☆		○ Yes ○ No
Summertime Puréed Banana with Papaya (Page 85)		☆☆☆☆☆		○ Yes ○ No
Naturally Nutritious Cantaloupe and Pear Purée (Page 86)		☆☆☆☆☆		○ Yes ○ No
Any Way You Please Chicken with Peas (Page 86)		☆☆☆☆☆		○ Yes ○ No
Tropical Chicken and Papaya Purée (Page 87)		☆☆☆☆☆		○ Yes ○ No
Growing Strong Beef and Potato Purée (Page 87)		☆☆☆☆☆		○ Yes ○ No
Beef and Carrot Purée (Page 88)		☆☆☆☆☆		○ Yes ○ No
Creamy Turkey and Spinach (Page 88)		☆☆☆☆☆		○ Yes ○ No
TEN MONTHS				
Scrambling for More Egg and Cheese (Page 91)		☆☆☆☆☆		○ Yes ○ No
Gotta Love 'em Lentils (Page 91)		☆☆☆☆☆		○ Yes ○ No
Lentil and Banana Mash (Page 92)		☆☆☆☆☆		○ Yes ○ No

RECIPE	DATE MADE	BABY STAR RATING (FILL IN THE STARS!)	NOTES	MAKE AGAIN?
Crib-Rockin' Lentil Roast (Page 92)		☆☆☆☆☆		○ Yes ○ No
Naturally Nutritious Lentil Mash (Page 93)		☆☆☆☆☆		○ Yes ○ No
Finger-Lickin' Good Lentils with Potato and Cheese (Page 93)		☆☆☆☆☆		○ Yes ○ No
Dreamy Green Beans (Page 94)		☆☆☆☆☆		○ Yes ○ No
Wahooo! Split Pea Stew (Page 94)		☆☆☆☆☆		○ Yes ○ No
Creamy Apricot Parfait (Page 96)		☆☆☆☆☆		○ Yes ○ No
Steamed Cauliflower with Swiss (Page 96)		☆☆☆☆☆		○ Yes ○ No
Tofu, Cheese, and Scrambled Egg Yolks (Page 97)		☆☆☆☆☆		○ Yes ○ No
Top-Notch Tofu and Apricot Purée (Page 97)		☆☆☆☆☆		○ Yes ○ No
Hand-in-Hand Cabbage and Apple (Page 98)		☆☆☆☆☆		○ Yes ○ No
Five Little Finger Sandwiches (Page 98)		☆☆☆☆☆		○ Yes ○ No
Bubble and Squeak (Page 100)		☆☆☆☆☆		○ Yes ○ No
Red Light, Green Light Bell Pepper and Beans (Page 100)		☆☆☆☆☆		○ Yes ○ No
Veggies with Tofu (Page 101)		☆☆☆☆☆		○ Yes ○ No
Sweet Apple "Cream" (Page 101)		☆☆☆☆☆		○ Yes ○ No
Tofu Banana Extravaganza (Page 102)		☆☆☆☆☆		○ Yes ○ No
Wee One's Kiwi (Page 102)		☆☆☆☆☆		○ Yes ○ No
Ham and Cheese Pastina, Please (Page 104)		☆☆☆☆☆		○ Yes ○ No
Ga-Ga Graham Crackers and Yogurt (Page 104)		☆☆☆☆☆		○ Yes ○ No

RECIPE	DATE MADE	BABY STAR RATING (FILL IN THE STARS!)	NOTES	MAKE AGAIN?
ELEVEN MONTHS				
White Beans with Dreamy Creamy Spinach (Page 107)		☆☆☆☆☆		○ Yes ○ No
Baby's Favorite Broccoli and Beans (Page 107)		☆☆☆☆☆		○ Yes ○ No
Black Beans, Avocado, and Yogurt, Oh My! (Page 108)		☆☆☆☆☆		○ Yes ○ No
Black Beans and Rice, Sounds Nice (Page 108)		☆☆☆☆☆		○ Yes ○ No
Pretty Please Peruvian Bean Purée (Page 109)		☆☆☆☆☆		○ Yes ○ No
Scrumptious Scrambled Egg Yolk with Cottage Cheese (Page 109)		☆☆☆☆☆		○ Yes ○ No
Refried Beans with Cheddar Cheese (Page 110)		☆☆☆☆☆		○ Yes ○ No
Super Silly Fusilli with Zucchini and Carrots (Page 110)		☆☆☆☆☆		○ Yes ○ No
Baby's First Raisin Purée (Page 112)		☆☆☆☆☆		○ Yes ○ No
Baby's Second Raisin Purée (Page 112)		☆☆☆☆☆		○ Yes ○ No
Carrot, Apple, and Raisin Delight (Page 113)		☆☆☆☆☆		○ Yes ○ No
Yummy-in-My-Tummy Raisin Smoothie (Page 113)		☆☆☆☆☆		○ Yes ○ No
Super Simple Cooked Beets (Page 114)		☆☆☆☆☆		○ Yes ○ No
Beet, Avocado, and Pear Rainbow (Page 115)		☆☆☆☆☆		○ Yes ○ No
Perfect Polenta with Cheddar (Page 115)		☆☆☆☆☆		○ Yes ○ No
Elbow Macaroni with Peas and Parmesan (Page 116)		☆☆☆☆☆		○ Yes ○ No
Itsy-Bitsy Apricot Chicken with Couscous (Page 116)		☆☆☆☆☆		○ Yes ○ No
Tasty Tofu and Egg Yolk Treat (Page 118)		☆☆☆☆☆		○ Yes ○ No

RECIPE	DATE MADE	BABY STAR RATING (FILL IN THE STARS!)	NOTES	MAKE AGAIN?
Cream Cheese–Pineapple Finger Sandwich Fun (Page 118)		☆☆☆☆☆		○ Yes ○ No
Pineapple-Banana-Blueberry Delight (Page 119)		☆☆☆☆☆		○ Yes ○ No
Raspberry Kiwi Melon Cup (Page 119)		☆☆☆☆☆		○ Yes ○ No
TWELVE TO SEVENTEEN MONTHS				
Yummy Yogurt Cone Sundae (Page 126)		☆☆☆☆☆		○ Yes ○ No
Super Scrambled Egg and Turkey (Page 126)		☆☆☆☆☆		○ Yes ○ No
Stupendous Strawberry Tofu and Prune Smoothie (Page 127)		☆☆☆☆☆		○ Yes ○ No
Baby's First Rice Pudding (Page 127)		☆☆☆☆☆		○ Yes ○ No
Strawberry-Banana-Tofu Smoothie (Page 128)		☆☆☆☆☆		○ Yes ○ No
Baby's First Blueberry Bread Pudding (Page 128)		☆☆☆☆☆		○ Yes ○ No
Crunchy Fruit and Cereal Parfait (Page 130)		☆☆☆☆☆		○ Yes ○ No
Goldilocks' Porridge (Page 130)		☆☆☆☆☆		○ Yes ○ No
Mmm Mmm Muesli with Yogurt (Page 131)		☆☆☆☆☆		○ Yes ○ No
Strawberry-Blueberry-Tofu Smoothie (Page 131)		☆☆☆☆☆		○ Yes ○ No
Winnie the Pooh's Favorite Breakfast (Page 132)		☆☆☆☆☆		○ Yes ○ No
Honey Butter (Page 132)		☆☆☆☆☆		○ Yes ○ No
Baby's Best Banana Buttermilk Pancakes (Page 133)		☆☆☆☆☆		○ Yes ○ No
Banana Split Cereal Bonanza (Page 134)		☆☆☆☆☆		○ Yes ○ No
Surprising Strawberry Omelet (Page 134)		☆☆☆☆☆		○ Yes ○ No

RECIPE	DATE MADE	BABY STAR RATING (FILL IN THE STARS!)	NOTES	MAKE AGAIN?
Cuckoo for Couscous and Raisin Purée (Page 135)		☆☆☆☆☆		○ Yes ○ No
Fruity Rainbow Breakfast (Page 135)		☆☆☆☆☆		○ Yes ○ No
Oh So Fresh Mozzarella and Tomato (Page 136)		☆☆☆☆☆		○ Yes ○ No
S-S-S-Smoothie! (Page 136)		☆☆☆☆☆		○ Yes ○ No
Wonderful Wheat Bread with Apricot Purée (Page 137)		☆☆☆☆☆		○ Yes ○ No
Tropical Pineapple Chiffon (Page 137)		☆☆☆☆☆		○ Yes ○ No
Mini Blueberry Muffins (Page 138)		☆☆☆☆☆		○ Yes ○ No
Nummy Nut-Butter Kisses (Page 138)		☆☆☆☆☆		○ Yes ○ No
Chicken Soup and ABC Pasta (Page 140)		☆☆☆☆☆		○ Yes ○ No
Stelline Stars with Cottage Cheese (Page 141)		☆☆☆☆☆		○ Yes ○ No
Awesome Avocado and Egg Sandwich (Page 141)		☆☆☆☆☆		○ Yes ○ No
Wonderful White Bean Soup (Page 142)		☆☆☆☆☆		○ Yes ○ No
All Dressed-Up Avocado and Carrots (Page 143)		☆☆☆☆☆		○ Yes ○ No
Luscious Lime Dressing (Page 143)		☆☆☆☆☆		○ Yes ○ No
Cheesy Potato Patties (Page 144)		☆☆☆☆☆		○ Yes ○ No
Awesome Asparagus Soup (Page 144)		☆☆☆☆☆		○ Yes ○ No
My Little Peanut Chicken Satay (Page 145)		☆☆☆☆☆		○ Yes ○ No
Perfect Peanut Sauce (Page 145)		☆☆☆☆☆		○ Yes ○ No
Super Quick Cup-of-Noodle Soup (Page 146)		☆☆☆☆☆		○ Yes ○ No

RECIPE	DATE MADE	BABY STAR RATING (FILL IN THE STARS!)	NOTES	MAKE AGAIN?
Toddler's Shepherd's Pie (Page 146)		☆☆☆☆☆		○ Yes ○ No
All Grown Up Chicken with Rice and Broccoli (Page 148)		☆☆☆☆☆		○ Yes ○ No
Lentils and Rice with Tomato Yogurt Sauce (Page 148)		☆☆☆☆☆		○ Yes ○ No
Baby Sliders (Page 150)		☆☆☆☆☆		○ Yes ○ No
Toddler's First Tuna Casserole (Page 150)		☆☆☆☆☆		○ Yes ○ No
Bok Bok Chicken, Noodles, and Carrots (Page 151)		☆☆☆☆☆		○ Yes ○ No
Flaky, Fantastic Fish Sticks (Page 151)		☆☆☆☆☆		○ Yes ○ No
To-riffic Tofu with Veggies and Peanut Sauce (Page 153)		☆☆☆☆☆		○ Yes ○ No
Perfect Poached Cod (Page 153)		☆☆☆☆☆		○ Yes ○ No
Marvelous Macaroni-Broccoli Sauté (Page 154)		☆☆☆☆☆		○ Yes ○ No
Benjamin Bunny's Carrot Purée (Page 154)		☆☆☆☆☆		○ Yes ○ No
Toddler's Favorite Teriyaki Chicken (Page 155)		☆☆☆☆☆		○ Yes ○ No
Tasty Tubettini with Peas (Page 155)		☆☆☆☆☆		○ Yes ○ No
EIGHTEEN TO TWENTY-FOUR MONTHS				
Summer Fruit Delight (Page 157)		☆☆☆☆☆		○ Yes ○ No
My First Avocado and Cheddar Omelet (Page 157)		☆☆☆☆☆		○ Yes ○ No
Pretty Please Pear Omelet (Page 158)		☆☆☆☆☆		○ Yes ○ No
Perfectly Plain Granola (Page 158)		☆☆☆☆☆		○ Yes ○ No
Aussie Smoothie (Page 159)		☆☆☆☆☆		○ Yes ○ No

RECIPE	DATE MADE	BABY STAR RATING (FILL IN THE STARS!)	NOTES	MAKE AGAIN?
Happy Hot Wheat Cereal (Page 160)		☆☆☆☆☆		○ Yes ○ No
Little Stars and Raisins (Page 160)		☆☆☆☆☆		○ Yes ○ No
Wonderfully Warm Grapefruit Crunch (Page 162)		☆☆☆☆☆		○ Yes ○ No
Nut Butter Delight (Page 162)		☆☆☆☆☆		○ Yes ○ No
Eggs Florentine (Page 163)		☆☆☆☆☆		○ Yes ○ No
Fabulously Fried Sweet Potatoes (Page 163)		☆☆☆☆☆		○ Yes ○ No
Ga Ga Granola with Yogurt and Berries (Page 164)		☆☆☆☆☆		○ Yes ○ No
I Want More Whole-Wheat Waffles (Page 164)		☆☆☆☆☆		○ Yes ○ No
Pleasing Pastina Breakfast (Page 166)		☆☆☆☆☆		○ Yes ○ No
Date Sunrise Surprise (Page 166)		☆☆☆☆☆		○ Yes ○ No
Super Stuffed Tomatoes (Page 167)		☆☆☆☆☆		○ Yes ○ No
Yo-licious Topped Yogurt Cheese (Page 167)		☆☆☆☆☆		○ Yes ○ No
Avocado in the Snow (Page 168)		☆☆☆☆☆		○ Yes ○ No
Emerald Nectar (Page 168)		☆☆☆☆☆		○ Yes ○ No
Carrot-Peanut Butter Spread (Page 169)		☆☆☆☆☆		○ Yes ○ No
Radical Rice Cakes with Almond Butter (Page 169)		☆☆☆☆☆		○ Yes ○ No
Avocado with Strawberry Cream Cheese (Page 170)		☆☆☆☆☆		○ Yes ○ No
Banana-Raspberry Dream (Page 170)		☆☆☆☆☆		○ Yes ○ No
Tuna Salad Surprise (Page 172)		☆☆☆☆☆		○ Yes ○ No

RECIPE	DATE MADE	BABY STAR RATING (FILL IN THE STARS!)	NOTES	MAKE AGAIN?
Stuffed Tomato with Tuna Salad Surprise (Page 172)		☆☆☆☆☆		○ Yes ○ No
Peanut Butter-Date Yummy Milk Shake (Page 173)		☆☆☆☆☆		○ Yes ○ No
Very Berry Smoothie (Page 173)		☆☆☆☆☆		○ Yes ○ No
Very Veggie "Meat" Balls (Page 174)		☆☆☆☆☆		○ Yes ○ No
Tasty Tuna Melt (Page 174)		☆☆☆☆☆		○ Yes ○ No
Popeye's Favorite Spinach Salad (Page 175)		☆☆☆☆☆		○ Yes ○ No
Wonderfully Warm Sherry Vinaigrette (Page 175)		☆☆☆☆☆		○ Yes ○ No
Cucumber, Shrimp, and Spinach Salad (Page 176)		☆☆☆☆☆		○ Yes ○ No
Creamy Lemon Dressing (Page 176)		☆☆☆☆☆		○ Yes ○ No
Yes, Yes, Yogurt Sauce and Eggplant (Page 179)		☆☆☆☆☆		○ Yes ○ No
Broccoli-Cheddar Soup (Page 179)		☆☆☆☆☆		○ Yes ○ No
Perfect Petite Pesto (Page 180)		☆☆☆☆☆		○ Yes ○ No
Starry Night Broccoli Pasta (Page 180)		☆☆☆☆☆		○ Yes ○ No
Rice, Veggie, Fruit Medley (Page 182)		☆☆☆☆☆		○ Yes ○ No
Tiny Tasty Chicken Nuggets (Page 182)		☆☆☆☆☆		○ Yes ○ No
Avocado, Cucumber, and Tomato Salad (Page 183)		☆☆☆☆☆		○ Yes ○ No
Happy Haddock and Tomatoes (Page 183)		☆☆☆☆☆		○ Yes ○ No

Index